1

Published by
Yellow Dog Publishing

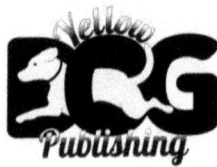

All rights reserved.

First published February 2024

Copyright © Brendan M Conboy 2023
www.brendanconboy.co.uk

Cover Design - Brendan Conboy

Printed in Great Britain
ISBN 978-1-7393684-5-6

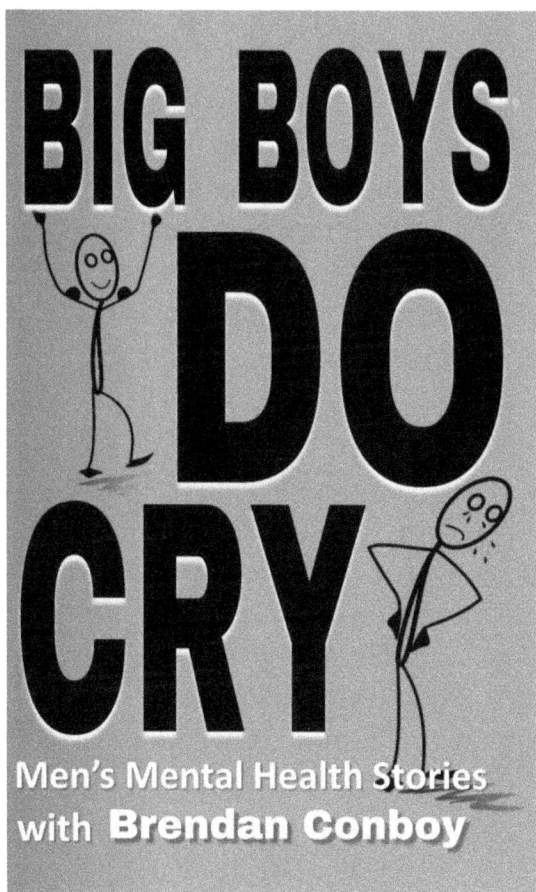

BIG BOYS DO CRY

Men's Mental Health Stories
with **Brendan Conboy**

"Yes, they do"

Brendan Conboy

Dedication

This book is dedicated to the brave men,
who found the courage to talk about
their mental health.

Asking for help and sharing the pain that you live
with is the most courageous thing you can do.

Also, to all men, especially:
The silent ones
The lonely ones
The still suffering ones
The recovering ones
The shameful ones
The painful ones
The unspoken ones
The broken ones
The rejected ones
The disrespected ones
The ones who want to die
The ones who never cry
The ones who believe the lie
The ones who would deny

That
Big Boys DO CRY

Thanks

Thank you to each of the story contributors.
It has been an absolute honour and privilege to
know these brave men.

They made themselves vulnerable
for one reason
to selflessly help others.

Without them, this book would not exist.

I thank God
for the gift of writing and storytelling.

Contents

Introduction: Mind Blowing

A survey of 1,000 men carried out by the Priory Group revealed the following:

77% of men polled suffered from common mental health symptoms such as anxiety, stress and depression.

40% of men have never talked to anyone about their mental health.

29% of those who haven't talked say that they are "too embarrassed" to speak about it, while 20% say that there is a "negative stigma" about the issue.

The biggest causes of mental health issues in men's lives are work (32%), their finances (31%) and their health (23%).

40% of men polled said that it would take thoughts of suicide or self-harm to compel them to seek professional help.

If you break a bone, you will not hesitate to seek professional medical help. So, why do we hesitate when it comes to our broken minds?

The human race is a remarkable collection of 8 billion beings spread over 57,268,900 square miles of land; each of us is unique. We are all individuals; even identical twins are not truly identical. Of course, we mostly have the same basic physical blueprint of two arms, two legs a torso and a head but there is far more to each of us that makes us human.

For example, it has been said that the human brain is the most complex thing in the universe. It has significantly more storage than an average computer, though a computer can process information exponentially faster than a human brain.

The average human adult stores 2.5 gigabytes of memory in the brain but unlike a computer, different types of memory are stored and transferred to different parts of the brain.

Our implicit memories are learned behaviours that we are unable to verbalise. They typically operate without conscious awareness and include our skills, habits and behaviours.

We perform these behaviours on a kind of auto-pilot, for example, tying shoelaces or a necktie. It's an easy task to do once learned, but it is very difficult to teach someone how to do it. I'm sure that there is probably a YouTube video nowadays.

Our implicit memories form in multiple areas of the brain. A key region of the brain called the 'basal ganglia' is involved in the formation of these 'motor' programs. The 'cerebellum' at the back of the skull also plays a vital role in the timing and execution of learned, motor skill movements.

In comparison to implicit memories, our explicit memories can be verbally expressed. These are memories of facts, events and locations. They can be consciously recalled and can be autobiographical, for example, what you did for your last birthday or conceptual, such as learning information for an exam.

These memories are easy to acquire. Yet, they can be easily forgotten, as they are susceptible to disruption during the process of forming and storing the information.

Our short-term memories are stored in the 'prefrontal cortex' but they are only held there for a short period. This is essential to the planning and formation of behaviours, ideas, and how we react to certain situations. The memory is then transferred to the hippocampus for our long-term memory.

So, why does this book about men's mental health include such a complex introduction to the workings of the brain? The answer to that is quite simple, we are all complex beings.

Many of us are never satisfied with who we are or what we are. Men can be especially competitive, it's a survival instinct from the days that we chased dinosaurs for food. Now, don't get me wrong, there is nothing wrong with a little competitiveness, it is what drives us forward to achievement and to better ourselves. What happens though when we are not as successful as we had hoped for? What happens when our perception is that we have failed? We compare ourselves to others in our competitive nature and see ourselves as inadequate.

Our minds cause us to question our own abilities. Negative thoughts of, "I'm not good enough" begin to overwhelm us. This is referred to as 'imposter syndrome.' It can be forced upon us by others, as they tell us that we will never amount to much. When people in positions of authority do this, such as teachers or parents, the damage can be catastrophic, if we do not have the cognitive ability to process the information with informed reason.

We hear expressions such as low self-esteem, low well-being, low self-belief, identity crisis, anxiety, depression, self-harm, disorder, etc. These are all labels that we wear and as we do, people make assumptions about us and our mental health.

As men, we want to be given more positive labels to wear, such as macho, handsome, intelligent, strong, fit, forthright, resistant, resilient, tenacious, successful, etc. This is not an exhaustive list and they are stereotypical labels. Again, they make assumptions but what happens in the mind if we do not fit this stereotype?

Is it wrong for a man to be tender, gentle, caring, compassionate, artistic, creative, supportive, etc? No, of course, it isn't yet, these are not considered to be stereotypical traits of a man.

When we do not fulfil our stereotypical expectations, does this cause conflict within ourselves? Is this one of the reasons why we have so many mind battles? Remember the competitive nature that men are stereotypically expected to have. We hate to lose a fight, so what do you suppose happens when we lose a battle in our minds?

The complexity of our mental health is such that I have never yet met anyone who can pinpoint the moment when they first started to be mentally ill, not accurately. We live in denial, not wanting to accept that something is not right. We become experts in camouflage, subterfuge and hiding our true feelings until we can take no more. Sadly, for some, the breaking point is so extreme that suicide is seen as the only option. Look at the actor, Robin Williams, no one was aware of the state of his mental health. He was a brilliant actor both on and off the stage. He portrayed a man with a happy life and full of fun, until the day that he could do it no more and he took his own life.

One of the problems with society is that we are

conditioned to think in certain ways, we call it our mindset. Western culture dictates that we keep a stiff upper lip and never show our emotions. We are nurtured with expressions such as, "Big boys don't cry" and as we grow older, we are told to, "Man up." We are perceived as weak if we cry in public and we are mocked for being different.

I want you to know that you can be different, you can break the mould, and you no longer need to comply with the stereotypical male traits. I, a fellow man, permit you to be yourself and to be the best version of yourself and I ask that you to also permit yourself to do that.

The stories contained within this book are examples of men who broke free from many of the mental barriers and constraints. They rose above the stigma associated with mental health. Not one of them has everything sussed, not one has cracked all of the problems, they all live with brokenness and are stronger for admitting it.

As you read their stories, gain strength and encouragement from them and use that strength to open up. Learn to talk about your struggles and to say, "It's OK not to be OK."

It's OK

It's OK not to be OK
To say, 'I hurt, I just want it to go away.'
It's OK
There is no shame, for your pain,
No blame, that is just the way
It's just the way
It's OK
It's OK to ask for help, to look after yourself,
Feeling lonely, left on the shelf.
It's OK because you matter.
So, stop the batter on yourself.
Life may be shattered and tattered
It's OK, just chatter, go on, have a good natter.
It's OK to say, 'I'm depressed, I messed up,
confessed my feelings,
my mind needs healing.'
My mind needs healing?
Is it really OK to say that?
Is it OK?

It's hard to admit, to submit, to commit
When you are in the bottomless pit.
That's OK, it's OK, You're OK
It's OK when you feel empty.
When your pain feels twenty,
times more than before

14

It's OK to say, 'No more' and roar.
Yes ROAR, cry out,
I cry out for those that cannot speak
It's OK when life is bleak to shriek,
or maybe simply squeak
When the road ahead is so steep.
And inside your head, you feel so weak.
It's OK, it's OK to pray, to say,
"God if you are there,
show me you care.
Free me from the snare.
See my distress flare.
Please answer my prayer."
It's OK to pray like that, to want life back.
It's OK to not be OK.
So long as you don't bottle it up.
It's OK to not be OK.
And to say that you've had enough.
It's OK to not be OK.
And admit that life really is tough.
It's OK.
It really is OK.
It's OK not to be OK.

Brendan's Story

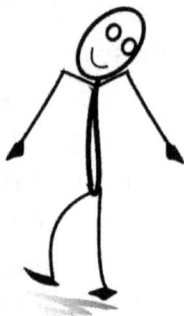

My earliest memory is at the age of four years old and my dad returning from the pub in the middle of a Sunday afternoon. Mum had prepared a traditional Sunday roast and tried to keep it warm in the oven but it had long since dried up. When Dad was drunk, he could be extremely violent and this was one such occasion. In his anger, he picked up the plate and contents, then launched it through the lounge window. The discarded meal along with the smashed glass landed on the front lawn. The neighbours heard everything but no one ever said anything; this was the way with domestic violence in 1964.

Our first seven to eight years are regarded as the informative years, they are the foundation of our lives and my foundation was one of fear; learning that violence was normal and to be expected. I, therefore, naturally grew up being violent and angry.

I remember that I lived my life on tenterhooks; with tension, anxiety and stress. I feared returning home, anxious that I might find my dad in a drunken rage. If he was out late and I went to bed, I would lie awake, wondering what mood he might be in when he returned.

By the time I was twelve years old, the fear had grown stronger and I was employing countermeasures; I slept with a knife under my pillow and I carried that knife with me wherever I went.

My life was full of emotional pain and distress. I had no control over the situation until I discovered a form of escape, a release from the pain. I can't remember the first 'accident', I think I slipped off a pavement and twisted my ankle. It wasn't a bad injury until something inside of me caused it to be so. At first, I simply sat on my bed and squeezed the point where it hurt the most. The pain was exhilarating but what excited me most, was that I could control it; I was in control. I limped to find a medium-sized ball-pane hammer in my dad's tools, this would become my comforter for the next few years. Sat on the edge of my bed, I smashed at my ankle, soft at first until the tissue went numb, then I would increase the force to inflict the maximum damage that I could resist.

Swollen and bruised, I would report the accident to my mum and later, similarly self-inflicted 'accidents' to my employer. I would tell the truth about the initial accident, but never disclose that the majority of the damage was self-inflicted. This was the early 70s and this was self-harm, though no one ever used that expression. I must have smashed myself up like this for at least five years and no one realised, not even the medical staff in the hospital (maybe they did). My mum would joke about how I was accident-prone. When I eventually stopped, I must have somehow pushed it to the back of my mind and forgotten all about it. I was in my 30s by the time the regressed memory came back into my mind and I admitted to others that I had once been a self-harmer.

Slowly and gradually, my mind devolved. Inflicting pain on myself was no longer enough, so I started to exert it on others; I became a bully. I went looking for trouble and found it at school and football matches. I wasn't that much interested in football but there was nearly always a fight to be had, especially if I went looking for one.

At the age of fourteen years old, my mind devolved to the lowest place; a dark, sinister place without hope. The ultimate level of self-harm is suicide; the final act of being in control – the ultimate release from pain. At least that is what I thought when I planned to throw myself in front of a train. I discovered something very important that day, in that dark place, something that has saved my life on more than one occasion; I learnt to talk.

On my way to the train track, I passed a phone box with a phone number in it for the Samaritans helpline. I dialled the number and cried my eyes out. The man on the other end listened. I don't remember what he said, but I do remember that he made me feel like life was worth living for, not dying for.

I was messed up mentally because of my dad, but a year after that phone call, when I was fifteen years old, Dad stopped drinking. The fear didn't go away immediately, I had to learn to trust him, which is probably why I continued to harm myself until I was eighteen years old.

I met a girl when I was fifteen years old and she seemed to understand me and accept me; she helped me to slowly sort my head out. Five years later I married her and three years after that we had our first child; life seemed to be positive. We had the usual problems with work (or lack of it) and money, the same as anyone, but something was missing.

In 1986, I discovered that what was missing was God and so on 5th May 1986, I invited Jesus into my life; yes, I became a Christian.

Some people may think that following that decision, life is a bed of roses but it doesn't work like that. My formative years provided me with a foundation of insecurity. I was still vulnerable and lacked resilience. So long as life remained even, without stress or curved balls, I could function well; and that is what happened.

At twenty-nine years old, I had been successfully running my construction business for three years. It had grown rapidly on the booming housing market, to the extent that I had employed twenty-seven workers. The housing boom was followed by a crash and I had nearly lost everything. Now, with a scaled-back team, my resistance was lower than I realised; it wouldn't take much to crush me.

The crush came in the form of a retaining wall that I had built. The wall was moving and required more structural reinforcement. I thought about it all of the time and I couldn't sleep at night. Sleep deprivation causes a person's brain to malfunction and mine was now telling me that I need to escape from this current stress; suicide was once again my answer. I now say that suicide is a permanent end to a temporary problem.

A train line ran past the wall that was causing me problems and I had the thought of jumping in front of a train again. It had been fifteen years since my first suicidal thoughts and the familiarity of feelings similarly overwhelmed me.

A memory in my mind triggered a learnt response; I remembered talking to the man from the Samaritans and how he had changed my perspective on life. I had to talk to someone but it would require an immense amount of courage, even more so than before, as this time the person that listened to me was my wife. It wasn't easy to start to talk but it became easier, the more that I opened up and I knew that she was listening; she understood.

Needless to say, I survived that mental episode, the wall is still standing and I am still alive. At the age of forty-five, I realised that I have roughly a fifteen-year cycle. I was no longer in the building industry and was working full-time for a Christian charity. I can't remember the exact details of what caused the stress and the mental overload; I just felt that I was at that familiar dark place once again; that place where suicide is my only option. My mind was already formulating a plan, a different method this time.

As before, my survival instinct kicked in, and my learnt behaviour to talk. Once again it was hard to do so but I am so glad that I did. I told my wife, not the details, the same as I am not telling you. There is no need to know the details, just the fact that I was in that low, dark place again. I shared my struggles with my wife again and also a counsellor friend who was also my line manager. I was so thankful and relieved to share the battle that was going on in my mind.

The three suicidal episodes that I have shared so far were milestones in my mental health journey. The were unbelievable moments of seemingly unbearable depression, but bubbling away between each of these events has always been 'imposter syndrome', that feeling of being inadequate, not good enough, a pretender. Other people believed in me, so why couldn't I?

I figured out that with my fifteen-year cycle, I would next be at risk around the time that I would hit sixty; however, it came early at the age of fifty-seven. I had been diagnosed with kidney disease in 2008 and I knew that one day my kidneys would fail and that I would require dialysis and a kidney transplant to stay alive.

In 2016, at the age of fifty-six, I started dialysis and it was hard. I fought on for just over a year until my mind broke. I won't go into all of the physical problems with my dialysis but I will say that I believe that it was my physical health that impacted my mental health and it still does. I had been on the transplant waiting list for eighteen months when I started to struggle with the fact that someone would have to die so that I could live; I needed a deceased donor. This thought rapidly changed into, "What if one of my own children had to die? What if they were to be my donor?"

It really was an unbearable thought and I started to think that I would be better off dead; everyone else would also be better off without me. For months anxiety consumed me every night as I cried myself to sleep.

I shared my struggles again with my wife (we all need someone to confide in). She told me to tell the dialysis nurse, so I did and was referred to a renal clinical psychologist and was prescribed anti-depressants.

I received a transplant after two and a half years of dialysis, over four years ago in 2019. I am still on anti-depressants and still feel that I need them. I often wonder how many people are on medication for their mental health and don't like to admit it. We are all unique, with our own journeys of mental health. I am sharing mine so that you can see the similarities and I hope that you will learn from them. The most important message that I hope that you will learn is the need to talk to someone whenever you are struggling.

Joe's Story

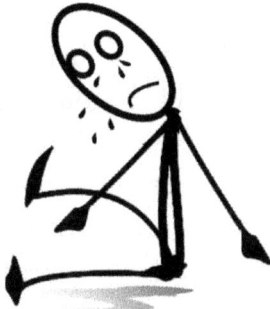

I'm 28 years old now and I think, as I look back at my growing up and my childhood, I wouldn't have said I had any kind of semblance of what it would be like or feel like when your mental health goes wrong as it were. For me, things just sort of worked, my brain did what it was supposed to do and that's it. I think, because of that, that sort of covered up and I didn't notice things that were perhaps slightly off. For example, my self-worth and my self-confidence weren't perhaps where it could have been. I wasn't necessarily making healthy choices but as far as my brain, it was working and functioning correctly. Yet, I was completely unaware that I could be making healthier choices. My teenage years were perhaps not the best foundation because of that.

Your brain just does what it's supposed to do until it doesn't and then suddenly you have to handle it and almost go back to the building blocks. So, I was at Uni and living in a sort of, do whatever I want world. I thought the world was my oyster and had a Devil May Care, throw caution to the wind lifestyle. I took a lot of drugs, mostly weed and nearly constantly. I had friendships with people who were taking drugs, those were the relationships that I was fostering at that time. It was very much a kind of echo chamber and we're all in this habit and lifestyle together. Then I had a particularly traumatic experience.

While high on a cocktail of different drugs... um, it's difficult to talk about, it's difficult for me to explain it because I don't really understand exactly what happened. I just know it was highly traumatic and I know it was a combination of what was really going on and kind of hallucinations. I had a heightened sense of all these things going on. I put myself in a dangerous position and then had this awful experience that I don't really remember like I don't recall the exact details. I know that whatever it was scared me and I know that whatever it was messed me up to the point of not being able to process what was reality and wasn't.

I think it's an interesting one and I've thought a lot about it especially because smoking marijuana has become more prominent and in popular culture, even as a health thing. The doctors that I spoke to after the incident, and doctors who are friends of mine, say it's quite a common cause of psychological problems for people. If you engage very heavily in it, then you have almost a persona and character that's yourself but also disconnected from reality in a sense. This was my experience anyway, I had a separate persona that I enjoyed, that wasn't really me, but it was a version of me. I liked that version quite a lot because I wasn't too worried about reality, my relationships or anything really. I was kind of purposely disconnected from stuff that perhaps I didn't want to face.

The doctor told me that I was definitely suffering from some kind of psychosis experience. It happened on two occasions. The first time was like a point of trauma and then the second time later having smoked weed, it happened again but worse. I was a little bit more aware of what was going on and completely paranoid. I had a paranoid fantasy that everyone was after me. I felt like this whole situation was rigged and genuinely feared for my life. Then I also started lashing out and was arrested, it was wild. The aftermath of that was just this complete drop and I was anxious about everything. I couldn't sleep because I was too scared, as my subconscious was going mad and my dreams were just terrifying. I couldn't sleep at night, so I had to sleep during the day. I didn't leave the house for a month, then I started getting depressed. It was like this sort of numbness, not like anger, not even pain or sadness; it was just sort of nothing. It was like a black cloud and I just desperately tried to stop my thoughts in my head, they were just too loud.

It was horrible - it was really horrible and I felt like I couldn't continue. My mind wasn't doing what it was supposed to and I didn't know how to fix it or what to do about it. That was the darkest point, I had the darkest thoughts knowing that I was having a psychotic episode again. The fear hit me as the last time I was a danger to myself and others. I couldn't control it, something could trigger it to happen again and I was really scared about that. I still had an irrational picture of my paranoid fantasy in my head and it was still quite strong. It's almost like fantasy and actual reality are in balance in my mind. That is what I believed and I couldn't trust myself. I couldn't trust anyone around me or anything I saw or heard.

I started to second-guess everything that happened and led up to that moment, I second-guessed everyone that I related to, like friends, especially those who had seen my first episode. It also didn't help that I hadn't had a very good experience in the hospital at that time. There was actual malpractice in the hospital so that didn't help me then.

So, that was the worst point; when I decided to seek help from Mind (a mental health organisation). I started having support sessions and they were really good. It wasn't too intense, if it had been I don't think it would have worked. I had the attitude of, fake it till you make it. It was basically, what were the small steps I could do to get back to where I was and we wrote down all of the steps, what they would be. First, it was just getting out of the house but going with people, then going out during the daytime by myself and then later going out at night. It actually helped me quickly.

I think I also need to say that faith is really important to me and it was quite key. There was a moment where some friends of my mum's prayed for me and that felt like a real breakthrough moment as well. It was a moment of hope that I needed to take those first steps when I really didn't want to. I had to step away from fixating on the worst possible or horrible solutions that I could take. Until that prayer, I didn't have a way back at that point but it provided a moment of hope followed by successful first steps.

So, I was getting back to a healthy place or at least a place where I was before any of the psychotic episodes, then came the realisation, that my lifestyle choices weren't healthy. I realised that discipline can be helpful and I wasn't living my life with purpose or doing things that brought me joy. I think the whole point of the crisis was helpful because it caused me to look at myself and my actions in a way that I might not have done otherwise. I do feel for people who have struggled with their mental health but never have that point of complete and deep crisis and instead go there slowly lowered into that dark place, it's a slower more gradual process. I feel that those people have it harder, rather than a sudden shock and a quick breaking point. I wouldn't wish what happened to me on anyone but it was a sudden wake-up call and I haven't had any sort of ongoing mental health struggles at all, which is fantastic. I feel quite free of it but I'm also much more aware.

Once you've experienced depression you can feel it creeping back in on occasion and then for me, it's like a kind of wake-up call to go out and meet with friends. Maybe I've isolated myself a bit accidentally or I've got too ingrained in work or something that I'm doing and I need to take a break and be with people. That helps me, it brings me life and energy. It can also be the opposite and I'm around people too much and I need to go away and walk in the country so I take two days to hike or go to a new city and just explore that. I've learned healthy habits and learned how to stay in control.

It's funny I haven't shared my story much recently, it's almost a past chapter of my life. I spoke with a few different youth groups and shared my story with teenagers who were going off to Uni. Those choices that I made are now on them and there are lots of very appealing things that you can do. It's very hard to be wise when you're 18 and you're away from your parents for the first time. I found that going in hard and saying that drugs are bad, don't go there, would be met with scepticism, like I'm one voice in a big noise, so better I think for me to encourage them. I encourage them to maintain connections with close family. I think that is important because, at the end of the day, it's those closest relationships, that could be family, could be friends, when things go bad, they may be able to support you. They may already have an idea of what's going on. When things go wrong, if you don't have honesty and openness, you're afraid to share with those closest connections.

Though I don't go as far as to say drugs are bad, I do say drugs alter your mind and your mind is your most precious thing and you take it for granted because it just does what it does until it doesn't. The choices we make have massive effects on our brains, so we should look after it in the same way we would any other part of our bodies. By taking drugs or drinking a lot or whatever it is you're doing, you are going out of your way to take control away from yourself and essentially altering this. However, much you think you know what you're doing, you don't, not really. For me, there was a lot of leaving too much to chance. That is the advice I give.

At Uni I was studying film and it was probably not the right choice for me. Another thing I would tell teenagers was, about their choice of what they will study. As for me, I really enjoyed the film industry, it's a bit of a hobby and I didn't know what else I would do, but it wasn't what I wanted to do as a career. Not surprisingly, I dropped out after my mental episode right at the end of the first year, there was no way I could manage to finish. After the second episode of psychosis, I had to do a spoken presentation and because I was in a group of three, I couldn't let them down. That was a moment I don't remember and I don't know how I got through it but I passed.

People don't think it's going to happen to them, they think they are indestructible. It's better to know that you have weaknesses and be humble about them, it's not a bad thing. I also think you can be confident in yourself while also knowing your weaknesses. That is better than just fully believing in yourself and you may be in for a nasty surprise; I suppose.

My life now is great, I'm married and that's a

very different life change in terms of mental health. I think that absolutely changes things, you have someone else whom you trust implicitly and you're bonded in a beautiful way. You have someone who you're able to share more deeply with than with anyone else, which is wonderful. There's also the work of maintaining that open connection, that doesn't just happen, you do have to put in the effort. When we don't, we have to talk about it and then we work on it. I think for both of us it's important to have that person that you're able to offload on and share in that way, where you talk every single day. You can check in and say if you're feeling a bit depressed, that is really beautiful.

You do have the extra burden of bearing weight for the other person as well and if stuff happens to them or if they're feeling low, you feel if something's not quite right in the relationship or you've miscommunicated or something, then you can take that upon yourself. I think that's quite a problem in men and is probably quite a common cause of mental health problems. I imagine relationship guilt and relationship breakdown could cause this. That's the balance between a healthy relationship and an unhealthy relationship. A good relationship has trust, that two-way thing and you can open up, but in an unhealthy relationship it just all goes inward, it all festers inside of us and then it explodes and gets out of control.

My life has now come to a point where I need some kind of change in my work life. I work in catering and have done so for ten years and I need some kind of fresh challenge, I'm starting to feel brain boredom. So, we're going away to Australia for a year and hopefully, that will be a time to enjoy each other's company but I'm also hoping that some ideas and fresh life direction start to emerge. I don't want to be stuck in a rut with the mundane routine of life, it can grind you away. That's the main thing that brings on my depression feelings. It feels like I am working to live right now and that's not really living.

Looking back, that whole mental episode was such an all-consuming chapter in my life. I'm grateful that I've been able to move forward, put it behind me, learn from it, grow and then live a normal life because, at that moment in time, I didn't. I wouldn't have believed that that could have happened to me.

Bramwell's Story

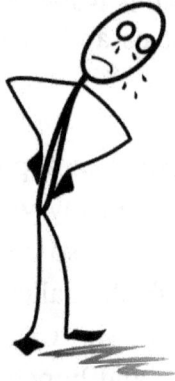

It's probably easier to start my story almost in the middle and that will become apparent as to why. Looking back to about 2013, I lost my marriage, I lost my family, I lost my house, I lost my job, I lost literally everything in my life and that was down to several reasons coming from one primary source, childhood trauma that I had suppressed as a teenager and into my adulthood. This trauma started to manifest itself in a way that affected everything and I was diagnosed with PTSD. 2013 sparked the beginning of the end of this life and in 2014 Jesus stepped into my life and turned things around in a way that I did not believe could be possible.

As a child, I was sexually abused by a male teacher. The way that he did it was the same as a lot of abusers. He befriended me, he showed interest in my education and I felt like he cared. He even started to buy me things and take me to places. I was a keen historian and loved my history and this teacher was a history teacher. This all came off the back of my home life which was okay, it wasn't bad by a long shot but my father was very busy with work and an Open University degree, as well as not being well himself due to mental health. My mum was very much the person at home who looked after us, she was a stay-at-home mum and she would protect us from the difficult moments at home. My dad taught me piano but he was very hard with this and whilst he wanted the best for me, he was like a strict headmaster at times. This history teacher didn't treat me like that, he showed care and compassion for me and interest. As he did that, he befriended me and started to groom me.

He would invite me around to his house, take me out to the pub and we would talk about history. I was 15 at the time. After being out we would end up back at his place and this was when he would start to touch me inappropriately and in turn, rape me. He then started saying, "You can't tell anybody, no one will believe you." This went on until I was 19 and I just felt like a little boy stuck in a bigger issue that I couldn't stop. The way that the whole thing would happen was the same every time. It was a similar scenario whenever we met, until one night I went around to his house, and as the whole thing was starting to play out again something within me told me, 'This has got to stop this can't carry on anymore.' So, I hid in his toilet and phoned home. I said, "You've just got to come and collect me." My mum came and took me home and from that moment he never contacted me again.

Following this I went to the police. My parents didn't want me to go, they had concerns about how it would all play out for me. I understood that but I still went, then I dropped it because I had so much pressure coming from elsewhere that I couldn't cope with it. I had a girlfriend at the time and the day after I'd run out of the house, I was going down to pick her up from university with her dad. I told him as we were travelling down and he was brilliant, he was so understanding. When we arrived at the university, we picked her up and I shared what had happened to me and she was extremely supportive.

I felt dirty and I felt like no one would ever want me. She was so understanding to the whole thing and despite having been touched by a male she still wanted to be with me so we ended up getting married. After about nine years of marriage, we came to a place where we were trying to help a friend of ours, who then opened up about childhood abuse to themselves. What then happened was everything that I had suppressed myself, came bubbling to the surface to the point where I was then having flashbacks. I started to get angry, I was lashing out, and I would hit walls and throw things. I couldn't cope. I'd have flashbacks of him and would literally be lashing out to hit him but of course, he wasn't there. The family home became absolutely horrendous, it was such a mess and a toxic place to be.

I went to the doctors and they diagnosed me with PTSD, so I knew where things were going. They said that I was going to live with this forever. I was put on medication and told I would be on this for my whole life. However, until this moment I had not realised that the choices I had been making in my life were coming from this childhood situation. I became addicted to pornography; I saw sex as love and so in a need for love, I would start having sex with other women. I got into swinging and my wife became involved as well but just with any addiction, the more I had the more I wanted.

One night, I ended up in a huge argument with my now ex-wife and she ran out of the house. The next thing I knew, I had the police on the doorstep and I'd been accused of domestic violence. I don't blame her; I don't think I could have ever lived with myself. I was not the man she married and I know that I was really horrible to be with. So, from that moment we were then separated. I was arrested, taken into police custody and the next day they released me on bail. I was unable to return home, as part of the bail conditions stated that I would not contact my wife at that time. They released me into the care of a female friend who was married but whom I also started having an affair with. A week later the police came back and said there was no evidence and therefore no charges.

However, my wife at the time had already been to court and got a restraining order on me. So, I couldn't go back to the house. I don't say that I blame her at all, I totally understand why she did it. So, I was now homeless for nine weeks. I continued to sleep on the sofa at my friend's house and whilst homeless, I continued to be the Head of Music in a secondary school, trying to maintain a job.

The Royal British Legion stepped in to support me because I'd done three years in the Territorial Army (TA). They helped me then get my own place, my own flat. The first night I moved in I literally had a mattress and a wardrobe and that was it, I had nothing else.

As I have already mentioned, I was already addicted to pornography, I'd use it to try and escape from everything, and then I started hitting the bottle. I was using drink, pornography and women to escape from what was happening in my head but also to escape what was happening in the physical. That was my life, that was the way it was going. I continued teaching but within my own head, I was now becoming more and more anxious and more and more unstable. My ex-wife moved a new guy into the marital home, with my children, the day after I was arrested and this created more issues for me with my mental health. I was like a time bomb waiting to go off and now and again I would explode, more often than not towards the new boyfriend.

I went back to the doctor and was signed off work. This though gave me more time on my hands and I also started to get in with the wrong crowd of women. This led to allegations coming towards me. I was arrested on a charge of rape by somebody who was a friend of my ex-wife and also a friend of my ex-wife's new boyfriend. The rape didn't happen but this woman had a track record of calling out rape and accusations. Thankfully, it never went anywhere, the Crown Prosecution Service (CPS) said, there were no grounds for a court case.

Within all of this, my mental health had spiraled totally out of control and I was using everything I possibly could to shut it down. With the arrests, my anxiety went through the roof. I was scared! I was living in a top-floor flat and the only way that people could get to me was by buzzing the door. I was petrified of that door. I was scared of going outside of it. I was scared of someone knocking on it. I shut down totally. It was then that I realized, I could not do anything myself to stop what was going on in my mind and so the night came when I just broke; but broke for the better.

I woke up one night on the bathroom floor and realised I had drunk a bottle of whiskey and I just cried out and said, "Lord if you are real, you are gonna have to save me."

I then heard an audible voice saying, "Trust me."

In that moment, He took away the desire to drink. He also took away all the flashbacks. A couple of weeks later from that moment, I realised that I hadn't taken any medication, not because I decided not to take it but because I had forgotten that I needed to take it. I had no repercussions from not taking it, I had no flashbacks and we're talking now nine years where I've not had a flashback. I've not been on any medication for PTSD since that day. The Lord healed me. He healed me totally, and in that moment, life started to change for me. I still had a huge anxiety and I still was addicted to pornography but drinking and flashbacks - all gone. I've always said that The Lord wanted to teach me something by taking that away but leaving the issue of pornography and women there at the time.

I had to walk through that, I knew that it was

wrong, The Lord had totally convicted me of it but the sinful nature within me just kept doing it. I went through counselling with a Christian counselling service in Swindon. I had a counsellor who was absolutely amazing and supported me brilliantly. She also helped me in regards to the fact that we were again going through court for the whole family case and Social Services were involved. I'd been classed as all sorts of things and all sorts of allegations were flying towards me and my life. That was when it came to the point where I couldn't do this anymore. I couldn't cope with what people were saying about me. I couldn't cope with this anxiety. I couldn't live with it. I couldn't live with being afraid of who's going to knock at the door next. That was the point where I was going to take my own life.

I took everything precious to me, my pictures and things. I put them all across my table and I took a photo of it and posted it on my Facebook feed. I just said, these are things that mean so much to me and there were pictures of family, pictures of my children and I was ready to take my life. I just thought I can't keep going. I had all the medication and had been to Asda and bought a large amount of alcohol. As I lay on the sofa ready to take all the medication with the drink the door rang and something that I can only now describe as the Holy Spirit made me answer that door. It was a friend of mine who I hadn't seen for about 18 months. He was baptized with me, he was ex-military, and I didn't know him until we were baptised. I opened the door and he said to me, "I just felt God told me I had to come."

He came in and saw what was about to happen. Straight away he knew. He picked me up and said, "You're coming home with me."

He took me back to his place and I was there for about three days. He and his wife were amazing. I poured out everything to them. They knew exactly what was going on. They told me that I needed to stop the relationship with the married woman, that she was never going to leave her husband for me and was spinning a story for me. It was just absolutely amazing how God moved through that situation. I even had an encounter with their dog Jess who I took out for a walk one day. Jess was leading me and she took me to a churchyard. What I didn't know was that in this churchyard was the grave of a baby that had been born to my friends. It was through this encounter that The Lord spoke to me clearly and when I told my friends, they said that Jess never went for a walk that way, they had never taken her. I was totally convinced that God was speaking to me in this situation.

Three days later I went home and they kept in touch with me. I then walked through a period of having to try and find myself, where I could be safe on my own. With all this stuff going on, social services, my ex-wife, I was feeling more and more unable, but I still was not having any return of the flashbacks or the desire to drink alcohol. This is where the counsellor helped because she started putting me in the position of the social workers. She would start to ask questions like, what are they getting told? What have they already been told? What have they seen in the past? It transformed me, it changed me because I could start to see things from another person's point of view and the Holy Spirit was helping me with that.

I was devoted to being in the Word, and from that my mental health started to improve. I got to a place where I was very happy on my own, happy to be sitting at home in my flat on my own. By this time, I'd lost my job, because I'd taken some extra time off sick. With the whole thing of the rape allegations the school were very supportive of me but at the point where the mental health was really starting to take over, they'd got someone else in to take my place. When I went back to work, they called me in for a meeting and the bottom line was that they just didn't want me there anymore. I ended up taking a payout from them and that was the end of my teaching career. I was then sat at home doing absolutely nothing, living off of what they'd given me but within that time, I was able to find myself. Over the next period of about three months, I had a spiritual advisor who helped me massively.

She started to teach me Ignatian practice, which at the time I had no idea about. The basic principle of it was to sit with God's Word and put yourself into the stories of Jesus. It was mind-blowing what The Lord did to me at that time. It was totally transformative because I could start to put myself into things. I remember one time she gave me two pictures of a nativity scene and told me to sit with the pictures and place myself into them. She asked the questions: "Where are you? What are you seeing? What are you smelling? I suddenly realised that this baby was born into this world and as a baby, had no power of His own, yet God knew the plan for Jesus. He was His own Son and He was God incarnate but within that, this same baby was the one who had called out to me and said, "Trust me." I started thinking, wow you actually want me for something and at that time I had no idea what it was.

I went on this journey then of, 'Okay the pornography has to stop. Lord, help me with this, give me the strength for it.' He told me that I would have to stand up in court and bear witness to Him and that was that. There was fear in that because it was like how, where, when, what? What are you going to put me through next? I just went through this period of seeking Him and seeking myself. Who was I? Who was Bramwell? I came to this place where I was comfortable with myself. I was comfortable about who I was.

Then, a friend of mine sent me a picture of a retreat at a centre on the Gower called, Nicholaston House. They said to me we really think you should go on this now. What they didn't know was this retreat was being run by Cath Woolridge and Sound of Wales. They didn't know that about three or four weeks earlier, I had been to an event with Sound of Wales, just outside Swindon and during that event, The Lord had healed me of anxiety. Throughout the whole night, I felt there was something that was inside of me which now I can say was a demon. It was inside of me and throughout the whole worship, of what the Sound of Wales were doing, this thing came out. I didn't do anything. I was literally coughing. I was trying to hold the choking back and it left me. By the end of the night, I was free of anxiety. I went to Cath afterwards and I had a couple of them pray over me. I explained what had happened throughout the night and these friends, who were now telling me about the retreat, didn't know any of that.

As soon as I saw that it was Sound of Wales and Cath running this retreat, I knew I had to go. I booked it up and the title of the retreat was, 'Knowing The Father's Heart.' What was even stranger within all of this; don't forget God has a plan for everything, was that it was through this that God would bring Natasha into my life.

Another friend of mine introduced me to someone a few years prior at 'Big Church Day Out.' They were from Swindon. We connected on Facebook but that was it. She was praying for me to be reconciled with my ex-wife. Once I had booked the retreat and the weekend before I was due to go, she put on Facebook that she was in Catterick, which was the army base where I'd done my training. So, me being me was inquisitive about why she was up there. I sent her a message and it turned out she was up there for her brother who had just joined up. We got talking and she suggested meeting for a coffee next week.

I said, "I can't I'm on a retreat."

She then said, "Oh, what's the retreat about?"

I told her the title of the retreat and she said, "Well I've taken next week off work. God has told me I need to take next week off but I didn't know why."

So, I said, "Well, do you want to come?" Now, I didn't know this woman at all. I had met her once.

Being the good Godly woman, she said, "Well if they've got a spare room then I'll go." So, she rang them and they had one room left.

In talking more after this, I said that it seemed silly for us both to go separately and so I offered to pick her up. On Monday, just a few days later, I parked the car and got out to greet Natasha. She closed the front door on me and I got back in the car. It was just like, this is crazy, what are we doing? We're about to travel from Swindon to the Gower together and we don't know each other. Thankfully, she opened the door and we both got back in the car and drove to the Gower. We still laugh today that when we got on M4, she said to me, "I'm South African and I've got a gun in my handbag." Well, that put the fear of God back into me. We got to Nicholaston House and Cath met us. She thought we were married; we had been talking so much and she said to us, "You are going to get married."

Little did we know that a year later we would be married and end up back at Nicholaston House on our honeymoon. Natasha, the woman I had met and had now married, was offered a job and we ended up moving to Wales but that's a whole other story. When I first met her on that first night at Nicholaston House, I sat with her outside and I poured out everything that was going on in my life. I thought this woman was not going to want to know me anymore after this and she said to me, "I asked God to bring me a man who would be totally honest with me."

I then had to go through family court but I had her by my side and we were in court for four weeks with all the allegations and everything. It was a mess but this comes back to where God said to me, "You're going to have to witness for me in court."

My ex-wife's team and particularly the social workers' team started to say that I lied about my PTSD, that I've never had it and that I've used it as an excuse. That was my cue, I said, "All I can say is I had it, it's medically there, you've got my medical notes, so you knew it was there but God has healed me!"

That was all I could say, I said, "Jesus has healed me. He's come into my life. He's changed me. He's transformed me." I was totally honest and open through the court case. They had to drop certain parts that they were alleging against me because if they hadn't, they would either say, God wasn't real or they would admit that He was real which they couldn't do in court. So, God was just moving through it amazingly. In the end, the

Judge summed up with what was quite a few pages. One of the things that stuck out was she said, "This man has fallen on his sword. He's been totally open about what he has shared. He has admitted his issues, admitted the things that he had done."

I had admitted the stuff where I'd lashed out, I'd hit walls, all of it, I admitted everything truthful and I stood against those things that weren't truthful but The Lord had taken me on a journey with my mental health. That journey brought me freedom.

Natasha and I got married a year later in 2017 and now I'm in a place where I have been restored with my children that I hadn't seen for five years. I've been restored with my ex-wife to the fact that we've all been on holiday together. It's gone beyond anything that I could imagine, from a place where I was addicted to pornography and sex and was having these flashbacks, to a place where now, The Lord has restored everything. He has brought me to a place where my mind is now. I'm not going to say, I don't struggle with anxiety and things at various times but I know that God is bigger than it and I can cast my cares upon Him.

Therefore, I've come to a place where, when I do have these moments, I've got a wife I can share it with. The Lord has given me two new children as well. We've now got Boaz who is two and a half. This was also after we were told we couldn't have children but The Lord had spoken to us both independently before we met and said, we would have a boy called Boaz. So, when we met and we shared this it was like wow.

When we were told that we couldn't have children, that affected me more than it affected her in a way. We ended up in the Bible College of Wales during the lockdown and a testimony of one of the lecturers was very similar. So, we walked out into the gardens at BCW and I laid hands on her stomach. I prayed Boaz into being and a week later she was pregnant. We were like wow this is amazing God has now given us everything. Since then, He's also given us a daughter. We were in the car listening to a biography of William Booth and the name Evangeline was mentioned. We both look at each other and say, "We're going to have a daughter and she's going to be called Evangeline." About six months later, Boaz was having a bad night. We went into his room and prayed. The

Lord gave me a vision of him walking with a girl and said, "This is his sister." The next day Natasha found out that she was pregnant. She's told me I'm not allowed to have visions from The Lord of any children anymore.

This is my testimony of what The Lord has done through my mental health and with my mental health. He has taken me through a massive journey. He's now given us a ministry that is called 'Wholeness Ministries' to see people come to Christ and be made whole and equipped for ministry. If He can give us a testimony, He can give it to anyone. If He can heal me of PTSD, which I was told I would live with forever, and anxiety and bring me through a suicide attempt, as well as bring restoration, I know that He can do it for anyone. I pray that through my testimony others can firstly be set free from mental illness but also that men can speak out about the struggles that they have and not feel ashamed. The Devil wants us to be ashamed of things we have done and wants to hold us in bondage but as Jesus said, "If you abide in My word, you are My disciples indeed. And you shall know the truth, and the truth shall make you free" (John8:32). He wants us to know the truth but it is only through His word that the revelation of the truth comes. Don't be afraid to share the truth, the truth of what you are facing because it will bring freedom.

James's Story

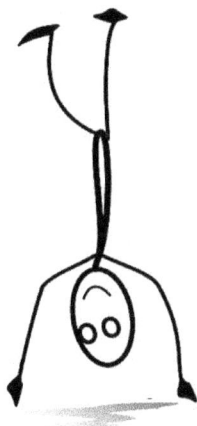

When I was 28 years old, I sat at my kitchen table writing letters with tears pouring down my face and onto the note paper. I knew that I had to see this task through and make amends.

The night before, I had visited a big Christian event; it was a Don Double Crusade meeting. On the way back in the car I just had an overwhelming sense that there was a lot of stuff I needed to sort out and put right; to at least begin to dismantle something, in the hope that it would get constructed into something much better. I can't remember what the guy spoke about but this was definitely the Holy Spirit saying, "Let's get on and get something sorted."

I was beginning to realise or surrender to the fact that I wasn't the guy that people thought I was, especially after being brought up in the Pentecostal Church. I was saved, baptised in water, filled with the Holy Spirit, and ticked all of the boxes but I knew in myself more and more that those boxes had been ticked for the benefit of other people; they weren't ticked for me. I felt I was a shallow kind of a person and I was aware that there would be a time when I would have to give an account to God. So, I thought why not do it now? Why not just be open before God by confessing and repenting? So, in a sense, I'm writing these letters to God; opening my heart in floods of tears.

For ten years I had carried some huge burdens which had crushed me mentally and I needed the weight to be lifted from me. There were three areas to cover – cheating, lying and there was stealing. These were the three specific things which troubled me, but I could justify them all in my own way. I'd say things like, "Well this is all right, it's not that much, you're okay, everybody tells me I'm okay."

I wasn't okay though, I wasn't happy with the

person I was; that I was pretending to be, the guilt was all-consuming. So, I dealt with the three things one at a time. To do with stealing, I didn't actually write a letter but this is the picture, if you like. I'm sitting there telling my beloved wife about all this stuff and bless her, she's standing by me and listening. I tell her that up in the loft, I have a box full of nice shiny electronic components. I was very much like a magpie; I was attracted to electronic bits and pieces and I'd had an opportunity to hive off with some of these bits from my employer. I had stolen these ten years earlier, when I was 18 years old and during those ten years, I had since left the company. I realised that the stuff was hidden away and I didn't have the means or the knowledge even to do anything with it.

I decided to contact the managing director of the company and said, I'd like to come down to see him. When we met, I told him what was on my heart and that it had been troubling me. He had time for me and was very gracious about it and recognised that this was a matter of conscience and conviction. The outcome of that was that he told me to go home, get the box and bring it back to him personally. He also said that once I had done that, I would be released from the burden, and I would be resolved from the responsibility. I was gobsmacked at that or I could say, I was God smacked!

I began to feel that this was the beginning of a huge release. I picture it like the story of the Pilgrim in the book, Pilgrim's Progress, as his burden was slowly removed; it was amazing, that rarely happens. I went home and went straight back with the box, it was a very humiliating experience. At that moment of handing over, there was a handshake and then I had a thought, this is God's hand; this man is representing my God. He gave me forgiveness and absolution; it was very special.

After that, I thought I never want to have anything in my house that doesn't belong to me, no matter how small and petty. I want nothing that isn't legitimate, it's a deceptive secret. I recognised that I tended to keep secrets and to deceive.

Regarding cheating, I had to write a letter about this situation. Once again, I did wrong. As an apprentice electrician, I was entered into a big competition organised by the Apprentice

Association. I had to wire up different junction boxes but also produce some practical metalwork; that was the part where it kind of all went wrong. The metal had to be fabricated using hand tools such as a hacksaw and file. It had to be made to certain dimensions and it didn't go well in that respect. I was persuaded to take a preformed piece of bar and file it down to remove any kind of marks from where it had been extruded, so that was a cheat. I also took more time on it than was allowed, then at the end, the other competitor's entries came into where I was working and I was able to have a sneaky look at what they had done. I picked up some extra points by making a few quick, last-minute finishes. This was all wrong, it was cheating.

Of course, the thing was, I ended up winning. The prize was an impressive sum of money and the honour of winning. When I went up for the presentation, the guy asked me how long it had taken me. I think he knew I had taken longer than allowed and that hit me. I felt instant guilt, but it was too late to undo what had been done.

Another awful thing about it was that I had my photograph on the front page of the local newspaper reporting my achievement. At the time I had proposed to my girlfriend and I said that the prize money was a useful contribution to my buying the engagement ring. So, after living with the guilt, I told my wife and she stood next to me, supporting me as I wrote the letter and my tears dropped onto the page. In terms of confessing and repenting, it wasn't just a sense of saying sorry to God, it was a case of repentance by actually, going to see people, to confess to people in authority. I didn't know where to send the letter, so I posted it to the Apprentice Association and also sent the money back.

Sometime later, I had such a gracious response from the Apprentice Association. They said they were sorry to hear that I had this on my conscience for ten years. It took me all of that time to reach the point that I just wanted to get it out in the open and deal with it. I would look at other people who were living their lives in a good way and I felt I was not measuring up, especially as a Christian.

I do feel that this was the Holy Spirit convicting me to make amends. I became a Christian when I was nine years old and baptised when I was 12. I'm not saying there's anything necessarily wrong with that but I was being carried along in a current and going from one stage to another and needed to find God for myself; to have that real conversion experience.

In regards to telling lies, this was a tax matter as I had lied on my end-of-year tax return. At the end of the form, I ticked the box that says, 'To the best of my knowledge and belief this is a true account.' I ticked that box, even though I knew it wasn't true. I knew that I hadn't declared some things. So, I wrote a letter to the taxman and delivered it by hand to their offices. I can remember posting the letter and thinking, 'It's gone, there's no turning back.'

Shortly afterwards I was invited in for an interview and the first thing the guy said to me was, "How did you know?"

He told me that they were about to take proceedings against me. I told him that I didn't know and that I just had a strong conviction about this, that I'd done a wrong thing. At some point, that taxman wrote a letter on my behalf and in it he said, "There is joy in heaven over a sinner who repents."

My first reaction was, hang on a minute, that's

not me, I'm not a sinner. Then I thought, well yes, I am, this is me; this is absolutely me. In every step of my repentant journey, I met a person in authority and it felt like they were representing The Lord.

My wife was thinking, hang on a minute we've got three young kids, and my husband's going to go to prison. She felt insecure, that we would be in big trouble. However, I didn't get prosecuted or go to prison. I had to pay recompense and pay what was due but essentially, I was forgiven.

This is my story of tears and it still makes me cry when I think about it. The sense of being forgiven is so strong, God's forgiveness is amazing. The temptations can still be there, and I still fight against that tendency to do wrong things and to be secretive. I don't want to go back to what it was like living with the mental burden of anguish and guilt, as it was for those ten years. I don't want to be that shallow kind of person. By God's grace, I was rescued from that and on the day of judgment, when I give account, at least to some degree, I can say to The Lord, "Thank you for dealing with those things."

Before these three burdens were removed from

me, I didn't value myself highly. It affected my self-belief and my self-esteem. I felt that I was a failure as a husband, a failure as a father and as a man. I remember that I once asked someone to pray about my self-esteem and as he prayed, he said three words, "It's alright son." I now think about how God looks at me and says the same, "It's alright son." Whatever I felt about being a father and husband and a man, I now realise that, I need to look at it in God's eyes and remember that I am His son and I am valued.

Dave's Story

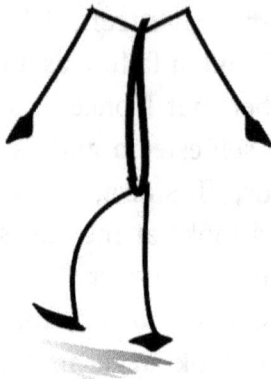

Like a lot of people, I think my first experience of
the dark cloud moving in over my life unbidden,
was as a teenager. I remember talking to my late
father about that and he told me that he had the
same experiences at that age and since I was very
much like him in a lot of ways that explanation
made sense, especially with the teenage
hormones. It probably never completely went
away but I didn't pay much attention to it.

Then in 1987, Dad had a bout of the flu and it
didn't go away. At first, the doctor thought that it
was ME; but it was depression. He worked for a
national bank at their head office. The bank had
a lovely scheme where, at the age of 60, if you
weren't going to get any more promotions, you
could apply to work for a charity and the bank

would pay your salary. Dad had a friend who worked for a charity and wanted to take him on, he loved the thought of this opportunity but it wasn't to be. The bank changed the system shortly before his 60th birthday and he no longer qualified. It was also the year of the so-called 'Big Bang' in the City, when financial industry laws were deregulated and he found that a deeply dispiriting experience.

He felt that a lot of the old moral values went out of the financial world and as a Christian that hit him very badly. I suspect that these were the two triggering events and he went off sick with depression and never returned to work.

That was the first diagnosis (in my lifetime) of anyone in the family with depression. Over subsequent years various other relatives also either had spells of depression or more long-term. I counted about five more of my relatives with mental health struggles at different times, including one who is bipolar. I still have my emotional ups and downs.

Early on in my Methodist Church Ministry in the 90s, I had some real problems. I walked straight out of college at the age of 32 into a terrible situation where I was looking after two churches. In the main church there were highly unsuitable children's workers and although the Children Act of 1989 had been enacted, all the safeguarding stuff hadn't come in. These people caused me a huge stress and in fact, for 18 months I lived under threats of violence. After two years the situation was resolved but it took a huge toll on me. I was still single at this point but engaged to a girl in the church and the next year that relationship went pear-shaped just before the wedding.

Put all these things together and it was just too much to cope with and I went off sick. I think some people thought it was just the breakup with my fiancée that did it but it was the straw that broke the camel's back after all the other stuff. My doctor signed me off for six weeks early on and during the first few weeks, I could not put a sentence together. I had a wonderful doctor but at that point, he was very careful to say to me that I was not suffering from depression. He told me that I was suffering from anxiety and stress and he persuaded me eventually to take beta blockers, which kind of gave my body breathing space to recover. Although it wasn't depression, it was on the way.

I came back from that and eventually moved on to my other appointments. I married in 2001, we had our two kids and started to notice that our son, who we've sometimes called mini granddad, was very much like my dad and me. As a child he had very dark periods, now at 19 he doesn't seem to have them and I'm so glad. I would have my dark times but my wife has been through a lot more traumatic things in her life than I have. She was only 13 when her mother died of cancer and things like that. She's always been the kind of person who says, whatever you're going through, just get up and get on with life. I couldn't hack it but she had a, just keep ploughing on attitude, and then we hit another really big issue.

Towards the end of my third appointment in the ministry, we were living in a town that the family liked. Unfortunately, while they were all happy living there, my appointment as a minister was a professional misfit and that is the kindest description. Some very awkward people made life worse. It was an appointment I shouldn't have said yes to. We did and we came to the end of the normal five years that you initially get appointed as a Methodist minister and I was a messed-up heap.

I didn't go to the doctor; I suspect if I'd gone then they might have given a diagnosis of depression. Instead, I used the Churches' Ministerial Counselling Service, a multi-denominational organisation. They work with church ministers and their families. I had a course of 12 sessions and I think one of the most helpful things about it, was that my wife and I are the classic case of opposites attract. I'm the geeky academic introvert, she is the practical university of life extrovert. The counselling helped in our understanding of each other. With her positive outlook on life, she couldn't understand why I was at the point of collapse over this thing and the result was that it brought us closer together.

We moved on to my next appointment and stayed there for 13 years. This in itself tells you it's a largely happier story. We had also moved to be closer to my mum and dad in their elderly years, as we felt that it wasn't right for my sister and brother-in-law to carry the burden alone. While we were there, first Mum and then Dad died and it was good to be on hand and to play a full role as their son but the dark clouds kept coming.

On occasion, there were clear triggers but not always. There was one definite trigger when some people were doing some shenanigans behind the scenes. This was a very small group whom my wife referred to as the coven. They were not happy that everybody else wanted me to stay longer and they tried to get me out. They made false accusations against me and that was a very dark time. It made me feel absolutely petrified because as a minister I have no employment rights. I'm not an employee I'm not even self-employed I'm what they call an office holder. I could have lost my work, my income and my home; it was incredibly scary. Fortunately, I had a boss who dealt with the situation very wisely and shrewdly but things kept coming and going.

Eventually, it was January 2021 and I had been having some real downers again. This time my wife suggested that I talk to the doctor; she understood me better now. Due to Covid restrictions, I didn't see a doctor face to face but I did have a really helpful phone consultation. He said to me, that it sounds like I'm someone who lives with depression. He told me that I've been living with this longer than I realise. That was an absolute, complete and utter light bulb moment. I mean, I think it would frighten some people to be told that they had depression but for me, the logical rational side of me could accept the explanatory power. This is the way that my geeky mathematical brain works. Now I could understand, not that I wanted to be depressed, I'd rather live without this but it was an explanation. It made such sense, what he gave me in that one sentence was so powerful for me. He offered me two things, to put me on antidepressants and the chance to do a course in cognitive behavioural therapy.

I asked if I could hold off on the antidepressants. I know medicines have improved, but in the late 80s when my dad was diagnosed, I remember him being on antidepressants and falling asleep by nine in the evening. I couldn't afford that with evening meetings as part of my work. So, I tried the CBT first to see how it went. The doctor gave me some links and I chose one of the organisations that does online CBT for the NHS. Sometimes I had a little bit of trouble getting my head around it but eventually, it settled into my mind and gave me a tool to ask questions in my head about a situation. It helped me to establish what is the truth here instead of catastrophising a situation. I have a special talent for that.

CBT helps me come back to reality. I don't mean that a switch was flicked and I was instantly better but I could start slowly coming up again. I had some trouble with it because when I was really down it was quite difficult to remember to start asking the questions, almost like I just wanted to feel the misery but ultimately, it's become a great tool. It hasn't cured me of depression, it's not something that can but it has helped me live better with it when it comes.

I think, as a Christian, I value CBT because it is an exercise in digging through to the truth and we value the truth as Christians, so that's good. Before I was diagnosed there were a couple of occasions when I preached, where I told people in the sermons about my dad's depression and that I'd had other family members with it. At that point, I was saying I've not been diagnosed with it but I have experienced times when a dark cloud suddenly appeared over my life. I found that received an incredible response from people. Some people say, Dave, we are so glad you've told us about that and that you as a minister can say that, it kind of helps us and encourages us in living with trials when you show your vulnerability.

I've shown my vulnerability in the past, not least during the rotten appointment, where I ended up in counselling and people just took advantage of it. If it helps people that is good. I recently published my first book called, 'Odd One Out' and I decided when I was planning the book, that this was the right time to go public on the diagnosis. When I was first diagnosed, I only told a select few people like my boss, ministerial colleagues and some of the senior lay leaders and they promised to keep it confidential and they did.

I was still nervous about how some people would react to me saying that I did have depression. I mean there is some bad Christian stuff around like saying it was a lack of faith, nonsense like you shouldn't have anxiety, you cast your cares on Him, all sorts of stuff like that. You get pushed down by some Christians for putting your head above the parapet and admitting that you've got a mental health problem; the Pharisees are alive and well. If you admit you have a broken leg that's fine, of course it is but mental health is just not seen in the same way. Society is starting to treat it better, yet there are still some very backward and judgmental attitudes in the church and that doesn't help.

I hope that my story will help others to cope when Christians condemn them for being weak. They shouldn't be like that. I've had people tell me that and how I respond depends on how emotionally strong I am at the time. If I'm in an emotionally strong place, I can respond to it and say that they don't understand this, this is an illness and it's a medical problem. If I'm emotionally depleted, it's much harder and if I'm not careful, I end up being very defensive. I almost have to watch what I say in case I say something unguarded and unwise.

A psychologist called Murray Bowen said, 'When you're in a conflict situation or you're in difficulty you need to look back at all your family of origin stories. What happened in your family that has contributed to the way you react?' Bowen suggests drawing a family tree and examining the relationships. Question how healthy each relationship was and what went on in them. I did some of this and it was a bit mind-bending and couldn't get my head around all of it. Later, an American Jewish rabbi called Edwin Friedman took up this family systems theory and said, we could apply this to institutions including religious institutions. He said, when there's conflict in the synagogue or your church, look at the origin stories of the church. I recently came back to this in preparation for starting my latest appointment.

I read a book by an American Baptist pastor, Charles Stone called, 'People-Pleasing Pastors.' All pastors are at risk of this. I found that Stone approaches this from a Bible perspective but he also quotes his particular interest in neuroscience. He approaches family systems theory and one of the things that he says makes you emotionally strong and ready to deal with the conflict is the questioning about the depression. Bowen called it our differentiated self. What he means is that you can within yourself, be emotionally healthy and strong and develop all that and you could have the compassion to connect with people but you remain differentiated from them. You just don't get sucked in so that, their emotions overwhelm you or become your reaction. He says that is an emotionally healthy thing to do. You have compassion, and you have spiritual and emotional strength but you remain different from these people.

I now watch myself thinking all the more about

whether and how well I showed that kind of level of emotional maturity. I think that it probably makes a difference in how I react. It's not easy though, it's not easy at all.

After a Sunday morning service and my first time at one of my new churches, a homeless guy came in wanting money. That is a tricky one and he knew how to press all the buttons. You have to have compassion but also differentiation to try and make the right response and that certainly applies to the depression thing too.

Tom's Story

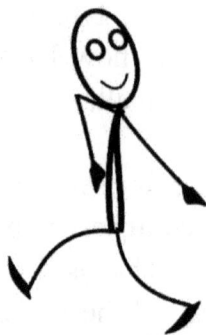

I was raised in a Christian home. My parents and grandparents are all very well known in the local churches. I always joke that I should have grown up as an ordinary middle-class white kid with relatively centre-right political and theological beliefs because of who my parents were, where they sent me to school and where I went to church.

On the surface if you looked at my life you would think this kid will turn out all right, he will be fine. I was sent off to private school when I was age 11 because I did well on a test. I was a nerd and if you put a test in front of me at 10 years old, I thought it was fun. Whereas, now I would look at it and think, I know what this means if I do well on this test, I'm going to spend the next seven years of my life being rampantly bullied, so let's maybe throw this test.

I didn't throw that test and therein was the beginning of my problem. I was in the church with a solid youth group, with two or three other lads who were in my same school year. There was also my older brother and his best friend and a group of girls who were the same age as me or slightly younger. Everyone got on and everyone's parents were friends. So, at the weekends, I had a solid unit of support and church family.

Let's start with the mental health issues, mine are quite serious. From the age of 10 to the age of 14, I was violently sexually assaulted by another boy. My parents thought that it would be good for me to associate with this kid. I will say at the time, I did not register just how much of it was sexual assault beyond my consent because at the age of 10, you don't have an idea of consent. So, when this kid sticks his hands down the front of my pants and then laughs, you think, 'Oh, that was a funny joke.' When he starts doing it once, twice, three times a month, for seemingly his own pleasure, that's when it becomes a problem.

One of the biggest problems was we were both at

the same fancy school. So, for seven days a week, for four years, I had to look him in the face. There was one full-on moment and there is no other word for it, it was rape. That only happened once.

By the time we were 14, I knew exactly what he was doing and there was barely any of it because I think he knew what he was doing was wrong. He'd gathered that much but it was almost like, he got such a kick out of it that he couldn't stop himself from doing it. As we grew older it became longer between events, then there was a six-month gap. The next time he came at me he realised I'd grown six inches and was half a foot taller than him. So, I bounced his head off a brick wall.

I've had some great therapy and I'll get to how that started later but I didn't tell anyone about this until I was 25 years old. So, I had 14 years of that but there was also other stuff that I needed to talk about.

When I was 13, my grandad, my mum's dad, passed away outside my old primary school. I had walked up to school with him, as I'd had a day off school because I'd not been very well with a 24-hour sick bug. He came over at half past three and asked if I wanted to walk up to the school to see some of my old teachers and pick up my little brother. I agreed and off I went. My grandad had had an operation two years before that I didn't know about. It was supposed to buy him six months. They patched up a rupture in his aorta and told him that he was weak and that if it ever happened again that would be it. They didn't think it would be long before it happened but he did live two more years. I never knew he was on borrowed time, my parents kept that from us completely. The teenage me thought that was a massive mistake but I look at it as an adult and wonder, 'What do you tell your 10-year-old at that point?'

I always think that if I had known he was on a clock, I think I might have told him about the abuse. I would have known I was on borrowed time to get help from my grandad, who lived at the end of our street. Grandad sat down outside the school and I went to find my younger brother. Shortly afterwards, I came running out with him and spotted a woman who was a nurse chatting to my grandad. She was also a family friend from church, whose daughter would later marry my older brother. She spotted me coming out of the school and knew what was happening. She was my mum's best friend and she'd figured it out. She attempted to grab us boys in the hope that we don't see anything. She grabbed my little brother and said, "Don't look, whatever you do don't look."

I'm 13, so yeah, I looked. I ran across the road sat down next to Grandad and I said to him, "You're okay. Are you gonna be all right?"

He said, "Don't worry about me pal, I'll be up in a minute." Then he just put his head on my shoulder and died, he was gone. At the hospital, my mum asked if he had come around in the ambulance. I told her that I didn't want to know, I was quite content that the last thing that man ever remembered was me and I'm okay with that. That one still gets to me occasionally; it was really rough and when you stack the other thing on top of that, it was tough.

Then a year and a half later my mum got cancer and my dad fell apart. Fortunately, my mum was okay. She had one operation and a bunch of radiotherapy and she was fine but I watched my dad fall apart for about three months. The family unit continued with church on a Sunday and you never would have known that there was a problem.

Then there was this other thing, my mum's brother disappeared off the face of the Earth after he had two kids. I didn't know he existed until I was seven when he got married. We all went to the wedding and I discovered I had an uncle. I got on with him really well until when I was 15. He had two boys and then he split up with his wife. We still don't know what happened to him but we know he's out there somewhere. He's still alive but he's gone. So, my mum was left caring for my now widowed grandmother on her own after the uncertainty of her brother being gone, then back, then gone again.

Then another shock happened. As mentioned earlier, I had three very close friends in the church youth group and I went with two of them on a church youth trip to Romania, running kids camps for a week and a half. When the three of us came back, we were told that Dan, who had stayed behind, had died in a sailing accident. A large boat captained by somebody drunk had not spotted his and his dad's boat and went straight over the top of it and killed him. The captain did eventually go down for it which felt like justice.

These are the things that have all impacted my mental health but I'm not done yet. At the fancy school, I was bullied rampantly. At one point I was locked in a bike locker in November. The school was on the North-East coast so it was freezing. I wore nothing but a school shirt, as they even took my blazer and trousers off me. I would have been in there overnight if it hadn't been for one of the caretakers coming to get his bike. I'd come around because I'd passed out but then I woke up. I heard somebody and I banged on the side of the locker and he let me out. None of the kids that did it were punished, not one. The ringleader was the headmaster's son who hated me for good reason.

The day after my grandad died my parents in their infinite wisdom decided to send us all to school. They wanted to see if we could get through a normal day, to see if we would be okay. As an adult, I look at it and I sort of get it but I'm never going to do that to my kids. I sort of get what their mindset might have been and my mum was probably dealing with enough. She was a daddy's girl and still is really. I imagine she probably spent the day crying at home and didn't want her kids there, which I sort of understand.

I was standing outside a physics lab when the daughter of the nurse who had helped my grandad asked if I was okay. Then somebody said, "He's just being grumpy, just leave him."

Then, the girl said, "No, Tom you may as well tell them, they're going to find out because your older brother is telling people."

The Head's son said, "Yeah, what's wrong with you?" He was making fun of me.

I said, "My grandad died yesterday, just leave me alone, not today. I can take your shit any day of the week, just not today."

He continued to wind me up, "Yeah, whatever your grandad's probably some fat bastard alcoholic in a care home."

I punched him on the nose so hard his head went backwards and hit the metal standpipe which was feeding the gas into the pipes and Bunsen burner taps in the lab. He cracked his skull and went immediately unconscious. When he was on the floor, I just started kicking him. I broke his nose, jawbone and cheekbone. I was dragged off of him by everyone and marched into the headmaster's office, which I now see as a massive conflict of interest. I was in front of the Head and he started screaming at me.

The Deputy Head had heard what had happened by this point and along with the Head's secretary came in. The secretary told him to stop. He told her to get out and she said, "You need to hear this, you will sit down and listen to me." I wondered what was going on. It turned out she'd just taken the phone call from my parents informing the school what had happened. She whispered it in his ear. I've no idea why she did that because I knew what she was saying.

The Head immediately softened and he looked at me. I could tell he was trying really hard because he knew I'd badly hurt his son but he looked at me and asked, "What did Joe say?" I told him and Joe was banned from playing rugby for the school for three years which was like his favourite thing. The Head also put him on Saturday morning detentions from 9 till 12 every Saturday for the next year and made him write a letter saying what he did. Three months later, once she was in a fit state to hear it, he made Joe go around to my gran's house and apologise.

There was a headteacher who knew how to make an example of his own son but obviously, Joe then hated me forever. He was wildly popular so that sealed my fate. If I ever thought the bullying was going to stop, it didn't. For the seven years, until the day I finished school, it was hatred from Joe, his friends and the kid who sexually attacked me. He and Joe became amazingly close friends.

With all of this stuff going on I shut down. I lied to my parents about everything. I was cold. I was borderline sociopathic at various points, in terms of my ability to never let it show. Like at church, anyone would think I was having a totally normal school experience. Nobody knew except the girl who had witnessed my aggression at school and my older brother, though he was at the stage of life where he wasn't going to fight my fights for me. He's apologised for it since and told me that he should have stepped in and done more. All the boys in my year really respected my older brother, it was a weird thing, they rampantly picked on me and because my brother never stopped them, they thought I was fair game.

I ran away when I finished school. The school

was all very set on getting clever kids off to university. It was all about the statistics. Don't get me wrong, I had some wonderful experiences there in terms of the music department and the few friends that I did have. I did loads of musical theatre, Shakespeare and things like that, that was kind of my little safe place. I started going to a different church and my whole youth group joined a Saturday evening thing that really helped when I was about 16. In that social space, nobody else knew my history.

I was already five foot ten and girls looked at me like I was, 'Oh, he's nice.' It was a complete ego reset in a way and I think I mellowed a little bit. Then I had a year of standard teenage relationships that worked and then didn't and then fell apart. I did some things that were wrong and so did they, but it wasn't incredibly traumatic. I had a girlfriend at one point who wanted to have sex with me. I did not want her anywhere near me because the only person who'd ever been anywhere near me like that was the kid who abused me. I look back at it and think, if the earlier stuff hadn't happened, I probably would have. It was a fearful response.

I ran away to Uganda. I went on a gap year with

the Baptist Missionary Society (BMS) instead of going to university. I cut contact with everyone, I could have very easily stayed in touch, admittedly it would have been once a week and it would have been emails, Facebook messages and video calls from the internet cafe place. It would have been easy to stay in touch on those days but I decided I was going to see who bothered to keep in touch with me. That was really helpful. I had this whole thing of telling myself that I would know who my friends were. I thought, that if I didn't bother keeping in touch with people, the people who really cared, would bother to keep in touch with me. I forgot that some people are more extroverted than others so what I actually got was the extroverted bunch of those people.

One of the people I stayed in touch with was somebody who I ended up dating for four years when I came back, it probably wasn't the best way to start a relationship, from a long distance. I had felt the need to stay in touch with somebody and she had reached out. I look back at it and think that it was not the smartest decision in the world and it led to some of my poorer life choices.

So, I came back and did a year at college followed by three years at university because amazingly when you're having trauma responses to everything and everyone, that affects your grades at school. I cruised GCSE exams on natural talent and then tried to do the same thing at AS level. On the AS level results day, I had the brown envelope in my hand with the head of sixth form standing in front of me. He knew what the results were but his face wasn't telling me. I thought he was standing there because I had done super well. I open the envelope and my stomach drops. Then I make a sort of nervous laughter, he thinks it's arrogant laughter and tells me I have nothing to be laughing about. Still laughing, I say, "I do sir, it spells DUDE down the page."

The joke carried on the following year when he handed me my A-level results and I said, "Call me a CAB." I had knuckled down amazingly most of that year. I didn't have a girlfriend so actually did some work. Despite all of the trauma in my life, I had actually done OK.

Recovery from trauma was a long slow process which started the month before I went to Uganda. We trained at BMS and I lived with everyone who was on all the different teams. There were some really wonderful people, we still go on holiday together and spend a lot of time together and go to each other's weddings and things like that. I immediately felt these people like me, I didn't mistrust them, I didn't think any of them were out to get me, and I didn't have a misgiving about a single one of them; so, they started my recovery.

Then there was the time I cracked in church. It was February 2019 and the pastor had only been at our church for a few months. I'll be honest I wasn't really paying attention until the pastor started talking about something quite interesting. I pricked my ears up, put my phone down and started to pay attention. He was telling a story and mentioned the '#MeToo' movement. He said, "I've not been here very long as Pastor but I want to set my stall out on that one just before I go back into my sermon. I need this congregation, this church family to know that if any of you have a '#MeToo' story, with me you'll be heard. You'll be listened to, you'll be given whatever time you need to tell that story, you will be believed and then you will be cared about."

I broke! I still have a slight reaction when I remember hearing him say this. I managed to pick up my phone, text my older brother who was sitting in one of the rows in front of me and I managed to say, '#MeToo.'

My brother turned around, hopped over the back of the row of pews on the balcony, pushed back past about six people and managed to grab hold of me before I started howling; it was a loud noise. Some people in the church have never bothered to ask me what the whole thing was about, because in church, when somebody has a visceral reaction over something, you don't ask but some people did. The following week someone said something along the lines of, "I heard a noise from upstairs and I wasn't sure who it was. When I saw you being carried out of the church through the door at the back, I thought, 'I hope he gets what he needs.'

Then they just said to me, "Are you getting what you need? If you don't want to talk about it, I understand, it's none of my business."

I said, "Yeah, I think I am now." I had sat with my brother and his father-in-law and wife in a side room and just cried and cried and cried. My whole body was shaking and it felt like all of it was coming out all at once. That was when my recovery really started.

.

Apparently, the pastor cut his sermon short, as he realised that somebody had reacted. From what I've been told, he quickly exited stage right and came tearing upstairs straight in the door and said to those with me, "You can go, this is my job." He's one of the best pastoral caring pastors I've ever come across.

The road to recovery

I chatted with my therapist about having my story and my name in this book. She questioned if I was doing the right thing. I told her yes, that more people should talk about this kind of thing. There are undoubtedly people like me out there who never said a word and at some point, somebody will read this and know that it all turned out alright.

When the pastor mentioned that I would be believed and listened to, the dam burst wide open and I remember making a noise. I have not cried like that ever. I had cried with a similar volume either in pain or at movies, to the point where I just couldn't move. My reaction now was a whole body heaving and sobbing, deep from within. My secret was out. I had never told anyone and the release with the physical reaction resulted in me being carried out to the side room. I remember watching the pastor's face. He had a look that said, 'This makes sense.' He hadn't known me for long, but he had known me long enough to suspect that something wasn't right.

You know that feeling when you stand up too fast and you have a head rush, I felt like that that whole afternoon and into the evening. The Pastor suggested that it was probably a good idea, while I was in the sharing mood, to go home and tell my parents. I knew that it would change my relationship with my parents for the better, so while I was being brave, I went to do the big scary thing. If I hadn't told Mum and Dad that day, I don't think that I ever would have. I would have told everybody else but I wouldn't have told my parents.

At that time, I didn't feel that I had a very trusting relationship with my parents. They both reacted differently to the news; Dad sat there dumbfounded and cried, whilst Mum wanted to commit murder.

A few years later, I saw my abuser at a festival. At first, I froze, unsure how to react. I ran to my dad to tell him and he hugged me, as if to say, 'It's okay he can't hurt you.' I didn't realise that my mum was standing not far away from my dad and she overheard. She started marching down the hill to confront the 'enemy' but Dad messaged someone and she was intercepted. It could have been a different story that day.

The next time that I saw him, sometime later, I think he was aware that I'd started talking about it. I had written a couple of things about it for my wife's blog and had made vague references but didn't say it was him. I was in town and he walked over to me out of nowhere. I was sitting in the Waterstone's cafe and he just pulled up a chair and said, "You do realise people think it's me."

I thought to myself, 'That's good.'

He told me that I couldn't write about him and I told him that I never said his name. I said, "There was no identifying reference to you! The fact that you think it was you, should tell you all you need to."

He has never made any real attempt to apologise for the abuse that he subjected me to, but as part of my recovery, I have moved past him. I'm not going to lie I still have days where I want to ruin his life, just for the hell of it because there is stuff, I will never get back.

My recovery has been a journey of milestones. The first was telling my pastor, then my parents and then my friends. Each milestone has made me stronger and when I met my wife, it was the first relationship I entered into being fully honest. I told her everything and that was another milestone. I said, "Just so you know, this is where I'm coming from into this relationship. It happened a long time ago, but I have an old scar that occasionally opens up, probably twice or three times a year. It's not pleasant, it's not nice and occasionally that might be a problem."

I am super honest about everything, not trying to cover anything up, not making excuses for not being willing to sleep in the same bed as her, because I was worried about waking her up with my screaming. My night terrors are probably down to once a month now. Sometimes I go a couple of months without them. When we were first married, it was a while before I woke in fear. My wife wondered if there was something she should be doing. She thought as we're married now, I shouldn't be having these. I had to tell her, "That's not how trauma works."

Seeing a therapist has also been another milestone. She has helped me to put together the pieces of my complicated mental jigsaw puzzle. She made me understand the need to apologise to my friends for lying to them. That helped to build the trust that I have with them.

Part of my coping mechanism is to talk a lot, but I don't do it when I am with my closest and most trustworthy friends. My therapist pointed out that this is not because I am relaxed; it is because I feel safe and she is right. I have now been diagnosed with complex PTSD and Emotional Rejection Dysphoria. This is where somebody could say something in a manner that is a completely ordinary tone and my brain will read it completely differently, to the point where I will think, that person can't stand me. For years I just thought people didn't like me, I thought I annoyed people. I thought other people liked me when they didn't or people didn't like me when they did. I'd read situations all wrong.

When I was at Uni, one of my friends was doing a study on people with Autism and she needed a control group. I said I'd do the control group test, but after the test, she looked at me and told me that I indicated as textbook autistic. I've never been officially tested; I don't want another label.

Another step to recovery has been to understand why I have what I have and how it links to my past. You are not born with mental illness. You don't catch it from others, it's not contagious as such, though to a certain extent, it is because we as people, like to damage each other. We may not realise it at the time.

My dad has this wonderful phrase that I find myself using when I train people in my job, 'Never make an accusation when you can ask a question.' I've quoted it in just about every job interview I've ever been in. They asked the question, "How would you handle this difficult situation?" My answer is always, "I would never make an accusation, I would ask a question." It immediately reduces tension and lowers the tone in the room. Even if someone is hopping mad, they see you as a person who is willing to listen to them. I was hopeless at this in my youth, but can now see how far I have travelled.

I have learnt to care for myself, it's a nice way of doing recovery; finding practical things to do to look after myself. I write off a whole evening a week where I say to my wife, "I am busy." Some of those evenings are sitting on the PlayStation chatting away to my friends in other parts of the world on the headset and shooting aliens and it's great. I think as a men's mental health thing, I will advocate to the ends of the Earth, to the women reading this book, do not disparage your partners who love gaming. You see them chatting away on the headsets, and you don't know who they're chatting to, they are probably chatting to other men like them, who are not lonely but who enjoy that sort of thing. If they were going off and playing football, they'd say, "Oh great they've got their football mates."

You can see women complaining all over the internet that their partner is ignoring them and playing computer games till silly o'clock in the morning. Gaming is a hobby; it is not an indicator that your partner hates you. This is part of their self care.

Vengeance is not a Christian thing, forgiveness is,

though I've had days where I want to just go out and ruin that lad's life. The realisation that vengeance isn't mine was the first step to that place of forgiveness. The second step for me was forgiving myself, forgiving myself for lying to everyone, forgiving myself for twisting myself in knots, for turning my life upside down, for the number of times I self-sabotaged. I could have a totally different life right now, I might not be married, but I might have been married several years earlier.

I think a lot of people would say that I'm fine because I never reached for the bottle or the needle. Comfort eating was a thing at one point and was probably the closest I got to any kind of addiction but I do say that I ruined my own life several times. I went on a mission trip for the wrong reason, I joined BMS World Mission for completely the wrong reasons. It led to some wonderful friends, but I didn't do as well at university as I should have done. I panicked and self-sabotaged!

When I got to the point of forgiving myself, it was midway through lockdown. It was 4.00am and I had just played 15 hours of a 'Destiny 2' raid (a computer game), as the sun came up. My bedroom smelled like a pigsty and I was a sweaty mess and I just relaxed. I remember the sun coming up and I had that Matt Redman lyric in my head, 'The sun comes up it's a new day dawning... Blessed be the name of the Lord...'

I remember having a moment where it washed over me and I thought, 'I'm okay, he didn't break me, I don't need to break him.' Then, finally have the thought of, 'I don't want to break him because somebody broke him more than I ever could, so I can forgive him.'

It had taken me 16 years to forgive him and weirdly the next thing that it gave me was hope. I opened my bedroom window because the room absolutely stank. I remember feeling like it wasn't just the smell going out of my room, it was a bit of me that I sort of let out of the window. I noticed the grey light of dawn and I could hear the birds singing. I was 27, in a relationship whcre I just bought an engagement ring and I had forgiven him. I was doing a job I enjoyed and I suddenly felt more whole; it had taken me 16 years.

To anyone who is in that place, whether you can compress it into six months or a year; that place where somebody has viscerally done something, that is their fault; it wasn't you. It's okay to take your time over it because if you don't, you will get to the point where you can't find a reason for forgiving them. Then, you can only conclude that it must be your fault. Somewhere, somehow, I think that's where a lot of people lose their way and they grab a bottle, they grab a needle, they stick stuff up their nose.

I'd love to say that I survived through faith. A lot of it was faith that I hung on to, I always had a group of Christians, God put them in places that I didn't expect to find such brilliant friends. Wherever I ran away to, God provided me with Christian friends. I'm now mentoring the 14-year-old child of one of the guys who helped raise me. That is the way that it should be. One-to-one mentoring is the way to go, it works, and it's the reason I'm alive.

George's Story

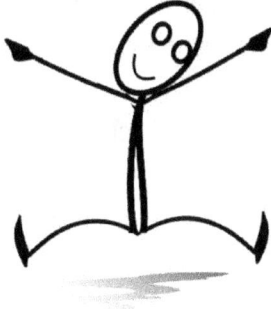

I suppose my mental health story starts from a young age. I was always different, looked different acted different and when you're a kid you don't think about it; you just go around and do what you do. From the age of about seven or eight, I was bullied for being different. I sort of managed with it and it didn't affect me a huge amount until the end of primary school, when I was age 10 to 11. I was making plans for the move to secondary school and then started to feel anxious. It was the first time that I would say that I was 'properly' feeling anxious.

I experienced seven or eight years of school bullying, most of the time it was name-calling, which turned into taking and hiding my stuff. One day, someone put my school bag in the bin and once or twice it was physical bullying.

There's that phrase people say, "Sticks and stones may break my bones but words will always hurt me" and that was my experience. It's the words that cut deeper than anything else and when you're in the stage of childhood and teenage years you're just trying to work out what life's all about, what you're doing and who you are. I think I already had some insecurities but when, pretty much everyone around you, tells you that you're not worth anything it has a big impact on the way you see yourself and anxiety grows.

*Editor's note: The saying that George refers to was originally quoted by E.H. Heywood in Boston, Massachusetts, on November 16, 1862. He said, "Sticks and stones will break my bones, but words will **never** harm me." Heywood said it to show that people cannot be hurt by unpleasant things that are said to them. This editor disagrees with Heywood and agrees with George, words can cut deep.*

To me, anxiety feels like water passing through your hands, you can't hold on to it. It gushes when it's strong and sometimes it's a trickle but it was always there, especially at secondary school, those years were tough. They say that anxiety is looking forward too far and depression is looking back and that generally speaking, was my experience. It's like something that you can't quite get a hold of, no matter how much you try. It runs away and runs circles around you.

People now tell me that I'm wise for my years and anyone reading this might think that, this was way back in my life but I'm only 23 years old now. To me, it feels like it was quite a while ago because I have moved on but it is still recent.

I still have the memories of depression and would say that anxiety caused me to feel depressed. It felt like I was stuck inside dark, dark, places. For me, anxiety makes me go quick and depression slows me right down, you can almost do nothing in a day and be absolutely exhausted because you're battling with yourself. That's the most exhausting work there is - when you battle with your mind. When you're depressed, and in that hole, it's like you're walking through treacle the whole time, physically, mentally, spiritually and emotionally.

I always felt like I was on the outside of stuff, I was never in a crowd, never involved in anything. I was the last person to be picked for games, most of the time in the playground or being bullied. That was my reality, the way it was and it wasn't until later in life that I understood that it wasn't normal, when I shared it with someone else, especially adults. When I started to share with them how people treated me and how they stole my things, they would tell me that it was wrong. I eventually started to think that I deserved this, I'm not worth anything. That was probably the main thing that my anxiety and depression centred around. Over those years, I had thought that I didn't have any words, my words were worthless, and I was obviously not worth anything. This is what I believed; it's horrible that people do that to other people.

I remember one morning when I was in my last year at primary school and someone at school had been threatening me. I just couldn't deal with it and I hadn't eaten any of my breakfast. Now, anyone who knows me will know that not eating is not normal for me, so my mum asked what was wrong. I just burst into tears and that problem ended up being sorted out by my mum. She went through a lot with me over those years. It's probably hard to see your child suffering the way that I suffered over the years, not just through bullying but my struggles and depression and anxiety.

I'd have days at a time I would just lie in bed and not go to school and not do anything. There were times when just the thought of walking to school or getting on a bus or the general thought of being inside school was too much. I couldn't get my head around it and that was at times when I wasn't being bullied at all; I guess I was school-phobic. I was probably school-phobic from the age of 11 until I finished school. One of my greatest struggles was the isolation and the more that I cut myself off, the harder it was and the more fearful it became to get back to normality. When I was 13, I had about three weeks off school, I was signed off by a doctor and referred to the mental health services for a year or two.

I had a really good child psychologist who helped quite a bit by simply listening and being there. Sometimes people want reasons that explain the way that they are, to put what they're thinking and feeling into a box and you know it's not always like that with mental health. My mental health has rarely been like that. Someone might ask why I am sad or anxious and I have absolutely no idea. There are things that you can't put a finger on and things that we don't want to put a finger on. It may be that I had a general feeling of uneasiness, periods of not being great or thoughts of going back to those places. Whenever you're on the up, you're always wary of what's going to be used to pull you down. You're looking around like one of those meerkats that come out of holes, trying to work out what could be the next threat and it's tiring.

My dad was a senior mental health nurse for 30 years and whenever he found out I was being bullied, he always wanted to take steps. He would want names, what they had been doing and which teacher he needed to speak to. He wanted to sort it, to find the solution, that's typically what men do and that was my dad's reaction to all of my mental health stuff. What are we going to do to get him better? He rarely asked how I was feeling, he just wanted to solve the problem.

Eventually, I was about 13 years old when I moved to a different school, which was a good thing. The bullying generally got a lot better, however, the problem then became school itself. School phobia still affected me. During my final year, leading up to my exams, I was only in school for one or two days a week most of the time. My attendance for religious education was 18% and I was stressed by the thought of exams. I thought it was like the end of the world but what I managed to do was to just focus on certain things, certain subjects. That was how I ended up with 8 GCSE passes including two grade A and two grade B.

That was probably the first real-time when I became aware of the power of resilience in the face of adversity. Every time before that, I had run away, got stressed, got anxious, and depressed. Then, I let it work itself out, that was my coping strategy before. Passing those GCSEs showed me how it's possible to be resilient and to have hope and that there is a future beyond darkened hard times. This was an invaluable lesson that I use all the time, anytime I'm going through something, I just remember all the times previously how I've got through things and it helps.

After school I started a catering apprenticeship with a not-very-nice head chef, he wasn't great for my mental health, he was another bully. Kitchens can be a difficult place to work, especially for a young lad who's just trying to learn stuff. I couldn't cope with it, with the bully, so I left after just three weeks. I stuck with catering and went to catering college but I was put on the lowest and most basic level. I knew all of the answers to most of the questions and the tutors tried to have me moved to a higher level but I had to stay. I was frustrated sometimes, but looking back on it, it taught me a lot of patience and resilience. There's a verse in the Bible that says, "Test everything and stick with or remain with what is good."

I think that's what I've learned to do, that's one of the things that has helped me over the years. In life, you go through lots of different stages and phases and lots of ups and downs and you hold on to good things. It was during that year of catering college that I met Jesus, well Jesus met me, Jesus found me.

I have been in dark places since becoming a Christian, especially when my parents split up. A year later I went to Brazil for the first time, for six months, then when I came back, at first, I had extreme culture shock. I had been in Sao Paulo seeing kids scavenge for food on the back of dump trucks and then came back to the UK and my friends were complaining about buses being late; that was heavy. It's difficult to fit back in, since I went to Brazil nothing has been the same. When I came back, that was at the time when my parents were selling the house, our family home that I had grown up in. Then, the week after we moved out, my nan died. I was already not great from coming back from Brazil and each of the bad things that followed was like stepping down a ladder, I just felt lower and lower. I stayed there in that depression for a few months and it was tough.

I think it was made less tough knowing Jesus but still tough. I often say to people, Jesus doesn't promise to fix everything, he promises to be with you and he was, always. It was made even harder because, at the age of 19, a lot of my friends were getting into drinking and drugs. When you're feeling crap about yourself and your circumstances and stuff, it was very easy to just get in the holes and stay in them for a time. At that point, I had another one of those times of questioning my worth. It's a question that I asked of God a lot. Why would you die for me? The answer is, of course, he wouldn't if it weren't for grace, in grace we receive a gift that we don't deserve. We've been given grace for us to show mercy, that is the difficult bit, showing love to others.

Some people might think that I am talking about my faith a lot but my mental health and my faith go hand in hand, I can't mention one without the other. A lot of the things that eat away at my mental health have to do with forgiveness, not forgiving ourselves and not forgiving others, not living as well as we should, and not loving ourselves; if you hold on to that stuff for long enough it makes you very bitter and angry. It does a lot worse for yourself than it does for anyone else but when we can let go of some of that stuff and give some of that stuff up, it's a process. It can take a while and you have to be willing but what I love about Jesus is he doesn't make us do anything. Often, in the Bible Jesus asked the disciples if they were willing. Are you willing to come after me, to follow me, are you willing to give this up to me, are you willing to forgive?

I think my mental health story and the struggles that I have faced have made me a nicer person. I am more compassionate and understanding and it makes me able to empathise. I don't like to use that word because empathy is about putting yourself in someone else's position but you can't do that, it is their position and it is impossible to feel the same as them. I prefer to say compassion because that's what Jesus had for people, in loving and coming alongside someone. When you're compassionate for someone, you're not trying to know exactly where they're at you're trying to be with them.

My experience has given me compassion, kindness and gentleness with people who are suffering. I have also learned that sometimes we need a kick to get us going. There were times when I was so depressed and gentleness wasn't enough. The times, when my mum came in and drew the curtains open, forced me out of bed and kicked me down the stairs, did help.

Now, when I have friends or family or someone I know struggling with these things, I use my experiences and knowledge to show compassion. It has shown me how to help others, that's what suffering has taught me.

I still struggle with focusing on doing things, more than I struggle with my feelings around the task. I used to not do things because I was anxious or because I was depressed. Now, I struggle sometimes to do things because of a lack of focus, not because of fear, anxiety and depression. There are moments when I feel some anxiety or some depression, but I wouldn't describe myself anymore as someone who lives with depression and anxiety. Yes, it comes up now and then but not anywhere near like it used to.

To any other young person that might be going through what I went through I say, talk to someone. A problem shared is a problem halved, talking makes it feel less, the burden, the weight is a bit less to carry when you have someone else alongside you.

My experiences have taken me down a path where I now live and work in Brazil. Through a community project, I work with children and young people who are at risk. I have also worked in a children's foster home for the last couple of years and intend to do more of that sort of work. I am hoping to specifically work with young men, probably young offenders, in the near future. I think I'll do this for the rest of my life, I don't really feel like doing anything else.

Tim's Story

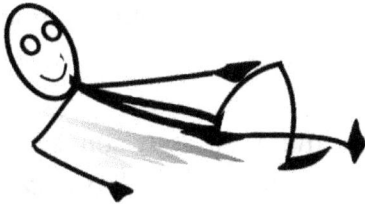

If you told me when I was a young guy, that I was going to publish four children's books I would have laughed. Yet, through my mental health struggles, I have grown to become more creative. I created a character called 'Paramedic Chris' and wrote stories about him. My time as a Chaplain to the real paramedics partly inspired me to write but it was also born out of my own mental health experiences, so this is my story.

There's that saying, "It's okay not to be okay" but I think people say it then struggle to put it into practice. There should be no shame in your struggles. I remember when I worked for the ambulance service chatting to the paramedic team, they said, "The mind's physical isn't it, it's all connected and when it's broken you get help."

I guess it's best to give a bit of a background first. I grew up in Norwich with three older brothers; my dad was a Baptist Minister. Those days were probably the best days of my life and my wife will kill me now for saying that. I absolutely loved my childhood but there were some traumas, bullying at school, which can affect you into adulthood. I've discovered how much it plays on your subconscious mind through counselling and the things that happened in childhood can come out in adulthood. I think one of the things, for me when I look back is that my dad's job meant that we moved around a lot. We weren't in one place for long, so it was difficult to settle down. That takes its toll on your mental and physical health and this background explains some of the reasons for my anxiety and panic attacks.

I spent eight years as a Chaplain and in my profession, people often opened up about childhood experiences. It struck me that there's something there in this and I realised people have hidden things. I know when I was bullied, I hid a lot of things and that caused me a lot of issues as well. I remember as a teenager walking to school and, in my mind, contemplating jumping off of a bridge and that's the only time in my life that I've ever thought about it. It was down to the bullying which I kept quiet about.

Going forward as an adult, my dad's last church

was in Dartford and I also worked a bit with the church and the youth. At the time I was doing a course with Oasis Trust in London, studying a bit of theology. I needed a placement and decided to do it with Dad's church, to do a bit of youth work. This was before I met my wife and we had some great young people there, which made it a great experience.

Then, I met my wife but shortly before we got married, one of the young people from the group was killed by a bus, it was extremely tragic. It was such a difficult time for the church and us as individuals as you can imagine and I remember going to see the family about a month after he died. They showed me his bedroom and his ashes and everything the way he had left it. I just took it all in at the time but a few months later I started to get some nasty, disturbing dreams about his death. I started to see images of his ashes and all sorts of different things. I started to shake and that was my first panic attack, though at the time I didn't realise and neither did my wife. We had no idea what they were, they were really crippling and it was because my brain was reliving and imagining some of what I had been told. It was like a type of PTSD.

I kept a lot of that in because I didn't really know what it was all about and I felt a little bit ashamed if I'm honest. I had just got married, 'I should man up' is what I used to say in my head; that's what I was thinking all the time. I tried to get on with life as normal, providing for my family and everything else but actually, I was trying to hide my true feelings and my thoughts. That just made it ten times worse, so I ended up going to counselling.

Counselling helped, so I thought that I could work through everything and cope. Then, on the first Sunday in 2010, the course of my life changed completely from a health perspective. I was having a lot of bowel issues. At first, my doctor thought that it was related to my mind, until I chatted to another doctor at church. This doctor told me that it sounded a bit more than that, so I went for some blood tests and discussed my symptoms with a consultant. They diagnosed Crohn's disease, I also found out that quite often with Crohn's disease comes mental health problems. Other sufferers that I know have also battled with different kinds of mental health.

Fast forward a few more years to 2019, I accepted a call to be a student Baptist Minister and it's quite a long-winded process as you probably can appreciate, you don't just go into that kind of role. Unfortunately, my dad was ill with cancer at the same time. At the start of the year, we were told he was in remission, so I felt it was right to just carry on with the job, that I was called into.

I was going backwards and forwards to visit my dad, who was two hours away from where we lived. We had moved house ready to take on this new role and then, all of a sudden, he rapidly deteriorated; it was a surprise to all of us. I kept going on adrenaline I guess, that's the best way of putting it and I didn't realise at the time. I can now see it in perspective, in hindsight of what happened. There was so much stress going on and Dad was dying. At the time I didn't see it, even though I worked as a Chaplain for the ambulance service. Often when it's your own relatives you don't see certain things you would see in other people.

So, I took the job on and we moved. I was inducted into my new role at a dedication service, a week after my dad had died. I did try to talk to one of the leaders to ask if we could delay the process, I wanted to say, "Let's just hold fire a little bit and I'll go lay for a year. I've struggled with anxiety here and I'm not great. I need to just slow down. Can we put the brakes on a little bit?"

They showed no concern and I felt that it had got me nowhere. So, I just decided to carry on because that's what happens when no one listens. This was quite significant because the Sunday after my dad died, I broke down not actually in the service but before the service. I'd walked into the church and they happened to be playing my dad's favourite song and that really hit me.

The lady in leadership, that I had previously tried to talk to, was quite a dominant character; she did not like that the minister was crying. I was crying. Her face and physical look told me that she wasn't happy. She was absolutely horrified and then a month later, I turned up to church prepared to chat about my feelings. She suddenly whacked me on the chest and told me to pull myself together. That, even to this day, has stood in my mind. I just couldn't contemplate why someone would say that. Okay, as a minister you need to be there and you need to look after people, I appreciate that but what's wrong with showing your weaknesses?

Actually, I don't think it is a weakness, looking back on it I think it's a strength, now that I've reflected on it. After that incident, there were meetings held and we had one that I would say was not a nice meeting at all. When I turned up there were two pages against me of things that I'd not done and I had only been there two months. During that time, I'd lost my dad and I was having, what I would call looking back on it, a breakdown.

I don't want to slag church and this is not what I'm trying to do but it gives a perspective. I think the church in general, particularly the Baptist system, needs more education with mental health and that's one thing I'm passionate about. Now I belong to the local Anglican Church and I have discussed this with the vicar. I don't blame the church for their lack of understanding. I don't want to put people off the church, that's not what I'm trying to do but what I want to see happen and I'd love to see happen is more education; not just in the church but in all walks of life.

Whatever role you play, whether as a man or a woman but particularly for us men, I don't think it matters if you show your emotions. I think you need to show them because, during my eight years on the front line in the ambulance service, I've been to people who have killed themselves. I've seen what happens when people have kept things in and that causes you to have a breakdown. Ultimately, because of the images in my head, because I've seen the consequences, I still don't feel bad about how I reacted; I don't feel bad about crying.

I have to admit, that I've seen people react differently, some people seem to carry on, other people don't. Also, unbeknown to me at the time of my breakdown, I didn't realise until a year later, that I was having kidney problems. My blood tests were all wrong at the time and it was a result of the Crohn's medication that I was on. When they took me off of that my kidney levels returned to normal. My mental health is still a challenge with anxiety but I'd say it's on more of an even keel. My story is an example that proves that physical can be linked to mental health as well.

I believe that people think, because you're a man, you're a dad, a husband and a minister and all that, that it's wrong to show your true feelings. There was this stigma and you might think it's just me saying it because of what happened to me there at that church, but it isn't. I've seen other people, in different jobs, treated similarly, where they're not shown any sympathy and understanding and basically, they feel they have no choice but to stop working. I still think there's a long way to go, I really do. You know people are struggling and they feel that they can't go on.

We are fortunate to have found a really loving church where I'd say we've had the complete opposite experience, which is what we needed. We have a vicar that is giving me responsibilities and rebuilding my confidence and I think that's what church should be about, supporting one another. I've been open and honest at this church about what happened, about my battles, particularly with anxiety. They still have faith in me and my family and that's what I think should be done in all churches.

Not just churches though, I even saw workplace bullying in the ambulance service and I see it in local schools. The list could go on but I'll say it again, the key thing is the need for education. It could especially help the person who's potentially making you feel worse. When I reflect upon where I was pastoring, I think people were probably too frightened of facing mental health problems. I discovered that one of the leaders couldn't cope with it because they had a relative in a similar position, they couldn't face any more of it. I don't shy away now from my battles. Why should I?

A panic attack, for me, is when I'm overthinking something; for example, I could be thinking I've got to do something uncomfortable next week. Anxiety builds up in my head, it's like a constant relay, I can't sleep and eventually, I hyperventilate. I avoid things and shake badly; it's horrible. From professional and personal experience that's what anxiety is, it's overthinking and fearing the unknown. When you evaluate it, it's not rational in one sense but at the time it feels like it is, it's so crippling and it's so awful.

Last week I had a panic attack in front of someone and it was over something quite minor. Now when I look back, I was fortunate because this person was very supportive. The week before that, I was in a different position, I was just dropping our son off at school and noticed a child was having an anxiety panic attack. Not everyone would be able to recognise it. I asked the mum if I could help and she accepted. I chatted to the child and was able to calm her down. When the mum asked how I knew what to do, I explained that it was a panic attack and that I also have them.

She looked shocked and said, "But you are really confident at talking and everything."

"Believe it or not it's true," I said, "it's a horrible thing, particularly for a child." I also went on to explain how it makes me feel and that in my own suffering, there's a purpose. It helps me to help other people. I didn't realise how much the parent respected me for that.

There really is a huge need for more support to be made available for anyone who is struggling with their mental health. One thing that bugs me, from a professional point of view is the number of times that I've seen this on an ambulance when I was Chaplain. A patient would be suffering a mental health crisis and we took them to hospital, then only a few hours later they are discharged. They need ongoing support but the system lacks the resources.

When I experienced the major part of my breakdown, there was such a long waiting list for help. I needed some kind of support and was fortunate that I was in a position at the time where I could go private. There are a lot of people not in that position and I look back on it and I feel for other people who are waiting they need support now.

The church needs to step in and help, I've said this in my sermons, not just in recent years. I've said it not just to do with my own struggles but I've questioned, what are we doing as a church. We need to do more, we're meant to be like a hospital in a sense, where we care for people. We could do a lot more to support people with mental health problems, even if it's just opening up churches more. The church we are at opens quite regularly now. We have meals on a Sunday afternoon, people can drop in and come and talk over a cup of tea and it's a safe place. We need to get that word across more to people. I feel that is what the church is called to do, to love and not judge. People are very quick to judge a person's mental health.

When I had my breakdown, it involved avoidance. I basically went into myself, so didn't go out as much. I was studying at the college in London and I started to not want to travel there.

I tried to avoid the anxiety of being with crowds and with people. I suppose it was also mixed with the grief of losing my dad. I felt very sad about my dad and saw repeated images and sounds of him dying in my head. I remembered what he had said towards the end. I guess it was a kind of PTSD, where you have the dreams and flashbacks, they came quite regularly to me and they're pretty scary. I didn't feel like myself, I cried and felt unworthy.

I questioned everything that I was doing. I asked, why am I like this? I told myself, I'm really useless and had all sorts of horrible, down, negative thoughts. I'm a useless dad, I'm a useless Minister, why would people come to me? I've never thought like that in my whole life but of course, this all came into my head and distorted my thinking.

The bully at the church certainly didn't help the situation, though, one thing that's helped me in my recovery, particularly recently is discovering that two of my predecessors went through a very similar experience and I think that's made me understand that it's not me personally. Hearing this has actually been part of my healing process, it's not nice hearing that other people were treated like that because I've been through it myself. I had to listen to people verbally slaughter me when I was in mourning.

I believe that my childhood bullying is also quite significant, when you're bullied and you have people picking on you, you try to avoid situations. I remember that on a number of the sick days off school, I wasn't sick. I feel that bullying hindered my mental health; any counsellor would agree with me. It's why I always ask my own children if they have had a good day; I ask them how they are feeling if they are okay. It makes you protective, as childhood bullying can cause long-term damage.

To stay sane now I use a journal, I like writing things down as it helps. I also do a lot of reading, and writing the 'Paramedic Chris' children's books. I've also been doing church things the vicar has me involved in quite a bit recently and told me I'm not finished with yet. The reason she told me that was because when I resigned, I was told, game over for you, you're finished with. I think looking back, for the person to say that was stupid, though I have grown through it all. I look back and think they spoke such nonsense, they're the ones that need to grow up and sort themselves out. I'm going to carry on with life now and be sane. I keep myself busy to occupy my mind, I think that's the key to mental health. To stop the vicious circle of negative and positive thinking and prevent the spiral out of control.

Another thing that helps me to stay positive is to encourage others. I am now mentoring others who are struggling with their own mental health, they seem to be drawn to me and I'm drawn to them. We're thriving on it because we're sharing our experiences and there's no shame in that. Our minds have been conditioned to see it as a weakness but it's not, it's a strength. When I understood that, I started to grow more and become more creative. I hope that my story will continue to help and encourage others.

Séamus' Story

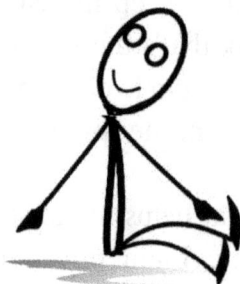

I'll try to start with a sort of an overview if I can and then maybe that will set the scene a little bit. I don't really want to go into my history or look back at my childhood but I have thought that maybe my upbringing wasn't the best. I'm 54, with two teenage daughters and I'm from a large family of six. I come from an Irish background but I've lived in England most of my life and in a way the story starts in 2002.

I met my wife and to use an old-fashioned term, we courted for three years and then we were married. We had the two girls quite early on in our marriage which is what we wanted.

Thinking back to my 20s and 30s, I suppose I never identified with having a mental health condition or concern. I knew that I'd suffered from depression and I was led to understand it was reactive, as opposed to clinical depression and I'd never had to use medication. I'd suffered several losses over the years and realised that I was probably prone to depression. It's not all to do with how your brain is wired, I think some of it is down to perhaps my upbringing and some unhealthy beliefs, including in myself.

I think that the trigger moment was when my marriage came to an end in early 2012. I remember it very well; it was the third of January and it's a day I can't forget. It's when my wife said that she wanted a divorce. That then, and in the two to three years that followed, was when my whole world was turned upside down. The divorce finally went through in 2014 and as happens to most fathers, my wife stayed in the house. I wanted my children to have stability and thought that was best for them. I suppose the divorce itself wasn't acrimonious, I mean it was actually quite straightforward. It was painful for me but there weren't really any disputes. I think, I just didn't want any conflict or anything like that and I just wanted to make sure my kids were okay.

I can't remember what the grounds of the divorce were exactly that my wife cited. It had to do with her struggling with my depression. She'd actually been very supportive in many ways and accommodating as any loving partner would be. They do as much as they can, don't they? Before the divorce, I did seek some professional help; I've never shied away from talking about things and I had some counselling. So, when we first separated, I asked that we have some mediation, not necessarily intending to get back together again, although that would have been my preference but more to agree on some of the practical things. Things with the girls and finances needed decisions. I suppose I needed a little bit of protection as well as I felt quite isolated.

Although I come from a big family, my family is quite fractured and, it's a horrible word isn't it; dysfunctional. That's a good description of my birth family, so I didn't have much moral support from them. I also felt they would have been upset and that it was a loss for them as well.

Following my divorce, in 2015, I went to see my doctor and was referred to a clinical psychologist. After two consultations with her, she said that I was suffering from something I'd never even heard of, complex post-traumatic stress. I'd heard of PTSD, I think most people have and like most people, I thought that's just something that happens to combat veterans or firefighters and police officers. Those people have suffered severe trauma like shell shock, injuries and death. What I learned from that diagnosis was that I'd suffered so many small traumas and losses which on their own are quite dreadful. The combination of these small traumas had developed to the point of breaking.

What happened to me in the wake of my separation and divorce, is that it triggered lots of other losses and traumas. These were compounded and they sort of built up on each other. Then in my divorce year, my mother passed away. That was quite traumatic in itself and then within eight weeks of her death, I also lost my job. I had been working for the local county council with quite a decent job but I just couldn't keep up with the workload. I saw a cruise counsellor and she explained with an analogy, she said, "You are like the boxer in the ring, you've had one punch, a second punch and then the third one just knocked you over and floored you." That's exactly what it felt like, I lost everything.

That was the year that I hit rock bottom, it was also the start of a sort of recovery. I was brought up as a Catholic and my mum and dad always took me to church. I didn't think of myself as religious. I didn't really feel I was living it and I think like a lot of young people I just drifted away and lost interest in the church. So, in the wake of my divorce, I felt I needed more. It wasn't that I needed religion or anything like that, not even church necessarily; I felt I needed a community of people. I needed new people around me; I needed a bit of a shot in the arm and I went along to a local church (not Catholic). It was the warmest welcome I've ever received in any church and it was fantastic. I've been to quite a few different churches, and different denominations over the years and never had a welcome like it.

I immediately enrolled in an Alpha course and I think that sort of awakened something in me. It allowed me to reaffirm my Christian vows, which is how my pastor phrased it. I thought that was a nice way to put it because he was honouring the fact that I was christened in another type of church. I'm a great believer in unity and because I grew up in Luton, I have a very multicultural background. I grew up with people from different faiths and cultures so unity means a lot to me.

I was baptised by full immersion, you know like the full Baptist Pentecostal dip in the water and that was incredible, it was one of the best days of my life. Obviously, there were other great days like getting married, with children being born, graduating from university when I was young, passing my driving test and going to America, but baptism was a special moment. It felt like it was the start of my recovery. I am conscious of framing my recovery in a Christian context and light, I can do that quite easily but because I work in a secular context, I try to break things down.

I've had time to heal from the marriage separation, divorce, losing the children, my home and my job but for any men and women, the part I think that hurts the most is the separation from your children. I think that is most painful and as a Christian, it doesn't make it easier. I don't feel I'm carrying guilt with me all the time but I do feel it's a massive deficit. It's the loss of the little things like just saying goodnight to your children, putting them to bed and things like that; it just broke me, it absolutely broke me. I don't know if any therapy could have fixed that and I thank

God I did turn back to my faith and revived it because I think it really helps. I'm not suggesting it's like a magic wand, it doesn't work like that. We're all on a journey and it definitely was a pivotal moment for me; going to the Alpha course gave me strength as did a charismatic church. I was able to see other people come to faith, some for the first time, others like me from different and diverse backgrounds.

This book is about encouraging men to talk about their problems but it's also about listening. When you hear other people talk about their lives it's humbling. That does give me strength, being able to sometimes carry others a little bit. It's not saying I've been through that so therefore I understand because everybody's formula for recovery is different. I don't roll like that but I think sometimes it's good to use that term, 'you walk with somebody' and I think that's very powerful.

I'm perhaps a little bit unusual generationally, my father was born in 1920 and I grew up with quite old-fashioned ideas. I perhaps, carried some of those ideas with me into my marriage. I feel that I've now become a little bit of a feminist since then, which is interesting but the point I want to make is I don't find it too difficult talking. I don't know if that's down to my temperament, I was very shy as a kid.

At the start, I mentioned that I don't want to talk about my childhood but I'm more than happy to talk about it. I was the second youngest out of six, with four brothers. Two brothers and two sisters were older than me and I have one younger sister. So, I often felt well protected. My mum and dad made me feel a bit spoiled even though by modern standards, we were probably quite poor. Still, I didn't feel poor.

So, we grew up in Luton, a factory town which was quite 'Londonised.' It was an interesting place to grow up because it didn't fit any mould and was very down to earth. My parents called themselves Irish immigrants, in my neighbourhood, everybody was an immigrant. So, I met people from all corners of the world. It was a little factory town but I could have been in New York, Miami or Frankfurt. My parents were from rural Ireland and we used to go out to the country a lot.

I was a very well-behaved kid, not rebellious, I was obedient. I loved being outside, I was always outside and loved to play football. As soon as I was old enough to walk, I was playing football and that was my passion. I was scouted by Luton Town Football Club but that didn't end well. I was injured and I couldn't play and my parents didn't want me to play professional football. Sometimes I can look back at that and joke about it saying I could have been one of those very rich footballers but it wasn't to be.

I had no childhood traumas or anything, just the normal things that go on in families like an uncle dying and things like that. I suppose my first trauma was when I was 21 when my dad died. I was still quite young and my mum had a bit of a breakdown. As she couldn't cope, she asked me and my younger sister to leave the home. That was quite traumatic first losing my dad and then having to lose my home. In a way, I never really recovered which is why I think, when I look back at the divorce, I can see the roots of my anxiety or insecurity in that first trauma. The word 'trauma' has become a bit of a buzzword and intergenerational trauma is something you often hear particularly in Irish families. You also see it in families where you've had maybe a father or grandfather or brother working in the military and I have that. My dad was in the Second

World War, and my brother and uncle were in the Army.

I didn't go homeless in the sense that I wasn't on the streets but I felt homeless for years after that. It probably wasn't until I was married that I felt safe again. That was probably the first time I felt that kind of security. So, there are days when I feel like I'm sometimes still dealing with the residue of that.

There's a Buddhist proverb that says, 'When the student is ready the teacher will appear.' My breakdown also gave me a bit of an opportunity to evaluate things and embrace the Arts, especially writing. Creativity is often birthed out of trauma.

Gary's Story

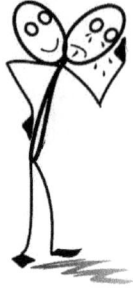

I'm 49 years old and have spent most of my life wondering who I am. I don't mean, what is my name, I'm Gary. No, what I mean is, what is my purpose? What is my identity? Where do I belong? These questions have led to much confusion in my life and I am only now, starting to understand. To help you to appreciate what I am saying, I'll start at the beginning.

Looking back to my childhood has given me a lot of insight which I didn't have as a child. My mother and father divorced when I was four years old. My older sister and I stayed with our dad and my mum left the family. We had a normal, well, as normal as possible, upbringing from there onwards with my dad.

We had regular contact with my mum and I grew up thinking that it was normal. I think my grandparents lived with us for the first couple of years. From Monday to Friday, I lost my dad because he had to work, so I felt quite lonely growing up. I put it down partially to where we lived, on a busy main road so I couldn't go out to play with other kids. Once I came home from school that was it, there wasn't any contact with other people and my dad often worked late into the evening.

I believe that this was the time when many of my insecurities developed. I remember (a lot) looking through the curtains to see his van. I waited anxiously for him to come home. Things weren't particularly great when he did get home but I felt lonely – an unpleasant anxiety. I did have friends at school, though even at an early age, they were mostly girls. I wasn't what you might call a typical boy. I didn't like playing football and 'rough and tumble' games. I was quite sensitive and I just felt more comfortable around females than I did around boys.

When it was time to go to secondary school, I sat the entry test for grammar school and passed it. The decision was made, I was going and I didn't have any choice in the matter. I didn't want to go but my dad had made up his mind. He came from a working-class family and was a working-class man but I think he had aspirations of being middle class and part of that was getting his children to go to grammar school, followed by a university education and a job that he could be proud of – to boast to his friends.

I hated every minute of grammar school, it was all so hyped up and academically focused. I wasn't thick, I had an average intelligence but I wasn't interested. I preferred more practical things like cooking and making things. The grammar school was only interested in high grades and how to achieve for the league tables. All their focus was on the top 10 or 20 of the class and everyone else was just sort of left behind, they were ignored.

The majority of the kids were from wealthy families and maybe a fifth of them were from working-class families that had scraped through the test. I kind of got on with everybody but I wasn't part of anything. From that early age, I felt like I was always tagging on to groups of people, not included, not in the middle of a group of people and again there was the girl thing. Although grammar school was an all-boys school, I had girlfriends from age 11 onwards, constantly, as soon as one finished another one would begin; I was never without a girlfriend. I didn't realise until I was probably in my late 30s that there was a big part of me that felt incomplete. I thought that another person's love could fill that incompleteness in me and make me feel whole. The incompleteness and emptiness were due to the absence of love caused when my mum left; that's where the empty hole began.

I scraped through secondary school, though I never felt like I belonged, I didn't like all the posh kids and I got on better with the 'Misfits,' the people that other people didn't want to be friends with. I didn't have any sense of who I was.

At home, my dad was very strait-laced, everything was black and white. He expected me to behave a certain way because this is the way to behave, without any explanation just this is how it is, this is how it's done, this is how you should be. So, I never really had any freedom to express myself and find myself. My dad could be intimidating, he wasn't aggressive or violent but he scared the crap out of us. We respected him, never went behind his back and we didn't answer back. He was sort of stern and cold, you just didn't dare misbehave because you didn't want to know what the consequence would be. It felt like he would see you as a failure if you questioned and we lived in fear, not fear of violence or punishment, it was fear of the unknown. I suppose there was very little emotion, he wasn't an affectionate parent, there was no praise, there was no enjoyment, he always expected better, there was always criticism and negative feedback, and there was never any encouragement or positivity.

At the age of 15 to 16, I didn't really have a clue who I was. I used to spend my weekends with my mum and that's when I started socialising and going to youth club and stuff like that. I did my GCSE exams and decided to leave school, I didn't want to carry on and that went against everything that my dad wanted for me. My best mate had been offered an apprenticeship with an engineering firm, so I applied and was accepted as well. I didn't have a clue what I wanted to do and I lasted three months, I hated being in a factory.

During this time there were a few big upsets, much of it is still a bit of a blur, but I ran away from home a couple of times. I'd have big flare-ups with my dad which led to me running away and I ended up living with my grandparents for a while.

I didn't realise it at the time but there were a few incidents where I self-harmed and I can't remember why. I thought up a scenario where I would cut my hand with a razor blade and make it look like I'd been attacked by a dog and then I would tell everybody. People would feel sorry for me, girls would be sympathetic towards me and comfort me. My dad would drop me off at school on his way to work, so I'd be there sometimes an hour before anyone else got there. I don't know why I went in early but there was one occasion that I do remember. I stood before the old wooden lockers with some of the doors broken off. I grabbed a door and I decided that I was going to break my arm and kept whacking the door on my wrist, to the point where I was in agony and then went to the hospital. I made up a story that I was pulling my bag off the top of the lockers and the door fell off and hit me. I didn't know what I was doing at the time, I never really knew and I certainly didn't realise that it was self-harm.

Somehow those incidents were buried in my mind for decades until I started coming through a period of depression that lasted about eight years. When I came out of that I remembered these things as I explored my past. By this time, I was in my 30s and things sort of clicked into place. With the realisation came a lot of confusion. I questioned why my 14 to 15-year-old self was hurting himself. I don't remember feeling sad or wanting something to change, it was almost a sort of subconscious behaviour.

So, at the age of 16, I left home and left school, that is when I started to experiment with drugs because all of my friends were doing it. I started by drinking alcohol and then tried Cannabis and LSD. I remember being terrified of drugs, as I'd grown up with the knowledge that Heroin was bad, so my perception was all drugs were like Heroin. Each time I experimented with something new, I was absolutely petrified that it was going to kill me or that I would become addicted to it. Despite the fear, I wanted more than anything to be part of something, to be accepted. I wanted to fit in but I still felt like an outsider. If I asked for a lift to the party, then I could go to the party but nobody was inviting me.

My search to fit in, to be wanted and to be loved

eventually resulted in a girlfriend becoming pregnant. Although we didn't have a relationship as such, I thought that it would be best for me to do the right thing, so I married her. Maybe a child would love me the way that I needed?

At this point, I feel the need to highlight that I have two younger half-brothers from my mum's second marriage. So, from the age of 10 to 20, I had baby brothers and I spent a lot of time with them at the weekends. For me, it was almost a lesson in parenting, like a practice run and I loved them to bits. I love my brothers, I enjoyed being there looking after them, taking them out and doing stuff with them. This is why I have always been quite open to the idea of being a parent. I hadn't planned for it to happen so soon, at such a young age of 18, but it would give me a sense of purpose, to know that somebody wants me, likes me and needs me. It rewards you. it makes you feel complete. This is why I embraced the idea of being a dad but sadly, it was another doomed relationship and we split up before the baby was one year old and she was pregnant again. That was a painful time, it was probably the most painful emotional time that I've ever been through, because I loved my kids with all my heart. I loved them, but I couldn't be with their mother. I had to leave and it broke my heart to walk away. To blot out the pain I jumped straight into another relationship, got drunk and took drugs; it was escapism.

After the breakup, I was diagnosed with non-Hodgkin's lymphoma, a cancer of the lymph node. I had the lump cut out followed by radiotherapy for three months. It completely wiped me out and I stopped working, I was just exhausted all the time. I'd wake up in the morning and go back to bed and sleep all day. Then when the treatment ended, they told me, "You're all clear, off you go and live your life." There was no thought that I might need to talk to somebody about what I'd been through and I was struggling both physically and mentally.

Sometime after, my ex-wife and mother of my kids announced that she was moving out of the area and that she couldn't cope with the children. They came to live with me and my new partner. The local authorities housed us in a flat and I thought that I had everything that I ever wanted. I had to stop work because my partner worked and didn't drive. My son was just about to start school and my daughter was about to start preschool, so I stopped work for two years. I was also drinking more, using drugs more and I was letting my partner do most of the parenting.

At that point, I felt that my mental health problems really started. It's when I began feeling the effects of it because I lost all motivation, I lost all desire, I'd lost my routine, I'd lost my purpose. I was a man, a builder, I went to work every day and then all of a sudden that stopped. For a long time, I thought that the trigger was me giving up my career. I thought it was the cause of my mental health problems, the low self-esteem and everything, but now I'm not so sure.

After the cancer treatment, I had a lot of joint pain in my wrists, they would just seize up and I couldn't hold a cup of tea or lift the kettle. The doctor prescribed me Amitriptyline and it turns out that, in higher doses, it's also an antidepressant. I was taking this medication for a few months and then I had a car accident, somebody crashed into the back of my car and I started feeling even more depressed. I'd never recognised it as depression before, I just felt like I didn't want to be here. I didn't want to wake up in the morning, didn't want to get up, didn't want to do anything, didn't want to live. By this time, I was married again, I had a loving wife and I couldn't tell her how I was feeling. I couldn't put it into words, I felt so sad, I couldn't vocalise it, couldn't explain and I felt guilty.

Mentally I beat myself up with thoughts like, "What have I to feel sad about? My wife's going out to work and all I have to do is look after the kids and make tea." I felt ashamed and blamed the car accident. I tried to claim through my insurance for damages to my mental health. The insurers did their investigations and they came back with the news that I had been taking antidepressants for up to a year before the accident and I hadn't realised.

What I now realise, is that I didn't always take the Amitriptyline and at those times, I believe I was in withdrawal; the symptoms are the same as depression. My circumstances didn't improve, things didn't get any better and then my doctor diagnosed me with bipolar and put me on another drug, Paroxetine. It didn't make me feel happy, it made things easier to cope with by making me feel numb.

The numbness took away other feelings, I didn't feel like myself, I couldn't laugh at a funny film or a comedian. I was devoid of feelings, then, as I would come out of the other side of it, I'd start socialising again, drinking again and taking recreational drugs again. I was full-on going to parties, thinking I was enjoying myself, believing I was happy, saying that I was better, yet leaving a trail of carnage behind me.

I used to go out, stay out all night, not come home and leave a partner with my kids. I was unfaithful, every time I went out. I went back to the doctors and found out that the medication side effects can be mania, promiscuity, risk-taking, and risky behaviours, it was absolute chaos. Then, my depression increased and I'd start substance abuse; it was a vicious cycle.

I could barely live, let alone do anything else. I was up and down, down and up and my partner wanted to move house. I agreed and we moved to the middle of town; it was fatal. I now had the choice of 10 pubs and I would drop the van off at home and say that I was just popping out for a pint. I'd be gone for the night.

I didn't want to be on the antidepressants anymore, I didn't feel like I needed them but every time I tried to stop taking them, I would have episodes where things would just go completely off the rails. This would usually involve drinking and drugs. The doctor simply told me that my manic behaviour was a sign that I was on this medication for life. I remember coming back home one Saturday lunchtime, after going out on Friday after work, crushing up my antidepressants and snorting them. I just didn't know what I was doing, I was on self-destruct. Eventually, my wife said she couldn't cope anymore and she left. I don't think I even realised for the first month, it was Christmas and I just bought a big bag of coke and used it over the festive season.

Within a couple of weeks of the realisation, I had a mental breakdown, that's the only way I can describe it. I wanted to die, I didn't want to face life, I'd messed it up and I'd messed up my kids' lives. Ruined everything for everyone. I felt like there was no going back, I didn't want to go forward, and I couldn't see a way forward.

I moved back in with my dad and my stepmum with the kids. I just wanted to sleep all the time, I didn't even want to be awake and the doctor came to see me. I wanted to be sectioned, I wanted someone to take me away but they wouldn't. They said that I wasn't ill enough to be such, so increased my medication.

My suicidal thoughts drove me to imagine and plan how I could end my life, though I never actually attempted it. I still had the responsibility of taking my kids to school every day, there were some days when my stepmum would do it for me but most of the time, they did force me to get up and out of the house. I didn't want to be here anymore but I didn't want the guilt of leaving my kids to deal with the fact that I had killed myself. So, the thought crossed my mind that we all go, it was a horrific thought to have but it seemed the only way. To leave them with the consequences would be the worst thing ever. It would be best all-around if I killed them as well. I can remember driving them to school and thinking, "If I swerve now that would be it, it would be all over." Those thoughts haunted my mind regularly for a month or so.

I later found out that Paroxetine is referred to as the suicide drug and in America, it's been linked to hundreds of teen suicides because, for the first two or three weeks of taking it, you feel worse than you did before. If you're already feeling suicidal it can push you even further.

I couldn't do it, I couldn't do it to my kids, they are my world and I love them. I decided to go back to my own house and my wife fought me several times for custody of the children and I always won.

I was still on a really high dose of this Paroxetine and felt like paralysis, I just couldn't do anything apart from the necessities. I got the kids up in the morning, fed them, got them dressed, took them to school, then I'd come home. I'd sleep all day on the sofa set an alarm clock to go and pick them up from school, feed them again, and try to interact with them. I would pretend that everything was okay and put them to bed. Then I'd end up sitting up all night, not able to sleep. This existence went on for about a year and a half. I had a mantra, "I hate my life, I hate my life, I hate my life." I couldn't get it out of my head.

I'd been single for quite a while whilst in this deep state of depression. I couldn't face being with anybody else and it was during that time that I read loads of books on mental health. I wanted to understand what was going on and soon I realised that this big empty hole had been created when my mum left. I'd spent my whole life trying to use other people and substances to fill that gap. I learned that I needed to fill that gap by loving myself, nobody else could make me feel better, I would only feel better if I could love myself. So, this sort of journey began.

It is hard to change your mental behaviour patterns and although I had the revelation of what I had to do; I fell back into another relationship. Once again it failed after three months and at that point, I said to myself, "I'm not gonna let this beat me, I'm gonna fight it, I'm not gonna stay at home." It was the hardest thing I've ever done, I forced myself to go to work every day and to keep functioning. I was working for an old guy called Bert at the time; it was me Bert and another young lad, Andy. I would not speak all day. Bert was a big part of my life because, through all of my ups and downs and months when I would disappear, he would always give me another chance; he seemed to understand me. At break time Bert and Andy would be sort of laughing and joking and I'd just sit there in silence, I couldn't communicate.

For me, depression is like having a metal helmet crushing your brain, trapping everything and pressure pushing on your brain; I wouldn't wish it on anybody, but I got through it.

I think that I had already come off of the Paroxetine and I started feeling everything again. Then, I heard about an art therapy course at a local medical centre. I don't know why but I signed up for it. It wasn't anything to do with art, colour therapy would be a better description and there was a lot of talking. Sometimes we painted pictures but it was more about colour and our response and feelings toward them. I connected with it and for the first time ever, started to feel like I was getting to know myself. I'd almost describe it as a kind of spiritual awakening, as I started to connect with nature, I'd walk around, look at the flowers and feel a warm glow. I could feel things again, I had self-awareness and it was cool. I noticed the world around me. I think I was just on the cusp of getting better when I met my next partner; she drank and did drugs every day.

By this time the kids had gone to live with their mum. I didn't have full-time responsibility for them anymore and we just embarked on this adventure of drinking and drugs, getting absolutely smashed every night. The kids would come over at the weekends and stay and after a few months, I thought, "I don't want to be doing this every night, I don't want to be drunk when my kids are around."

The relationship almost broke up and then she fell pregnant, so we decided to give it a go. I carried on drinking and using drugs a couple of times a week and it soon increased to three times a week; out of control again.

Then the lymphoma came back again and I had to have chemotherapy this time because it was in my abdomen. I'd had checkups ever since the first outbreak 20 years earlier. Now the consultant told me, the type of lymphoma that I have will come back every 20 years almost to the day. I could set an alarm; every 20 years it will come back somewhere else in my body. He calls it an inconvenience as it's one of the easiest to treat and one of the most successful to recover from; as long as it's treated it's not life-threatening.

This was like a wake-up call and I thought that I had recovered from the depression. I had a life of addiction but I didn't see myself as an addict. I still wasn't happy or satisfied with life, the more unhappy I was, the more drugs I'd take. We had another two kids but I still wasn't happy.

There was a point when I had been having acupuncture for about six months with somebody who specialised in helping people with their addictions. I wanted to change but I didn't see myself as an addict. I had a drug habit that I thought I could control, if I could use drugs once a fortnight or once a week then I would be okay. The acupuncturist suggested a few times about going to Alcoholics Anonymous and Narcotics Anonymous and I just shrugged it off, saying it's not for me.

My mind changed when I was at work on a bank holiday Monday. The customer gave us a bottle of beer at break time because it was a holiday and for me, alcohol always went with drugs. I had some coke in my pocket left over from the weekend and the next thing I know, I'm up in his bathroom snorting lines of the white powder. I think to myself, "What the hell am I doing?" It was a spiritual awakening as I admitted to myself, "I'm an addict, I have no control over this."

I rang the partner of the acupuncturist and said, "I'm completely powerless over this, I can't do it on my own, I need help." So, I started going to meetings.

Since the holiday Monday, my cravings were gone, I didn't crave it once, it was a miracle it was taken away from me. Then, after two months, I had a relapse. I think it happened because it hadn't taken any effort from me, all I had to do was acknowledge that I was an addict and it was gone, so I was a bit complacent. I had used the drugs with my wife and because of her, it caused us to argue, I started thinking, "I've been brainwashed, I've had all my choices taken away from me, and I've been controlled somehow."

The next day it felt like spiritual suicide, I'd had this spiritual awakening and my addiction removed from me and then I'd put two fingers up to it and tried to poison myself again. It took me about five days to get over that relapse. I was bordering on suicidal again, it really took me that low. The thought that I'd risk throwing my chance away, I'd been gifted this opportunity of a new beginning and when it happened, I couldn't even go out of the house, I was so paranoid, I hated myself that much, I couldn't bear to be around anybody. Since then, I've worked every day for my recovery. I thought that the substances took away all the stress in my life, but they actually caused it.

I've got a really good sponsor and I'm working through the 12 steps. I am finding out who I am, why am I like I am, why I choose to do the things I do and how can I live better. I've been clean for a year now and I've grown more in this last year than the previous 48. My life is mine now, I rely on a higher power, and that higher power can be the thing that you choose it to be. I call it God but to me, it's the universe, to me God is love; an energy. I believe in creation and that everything we see was created. I don't buy into the religious version of God if that makes sense but I pray every day.

Now that I have taken control of my life, I felt that it was best to move out of my marital home, so I have separated from my wife. She stopped using drugs at the same time as me because I was the supplier, so she didn't have much choice but she didn't engage in any program of recovery. She's still the same person she was the day she stopped; she's still messed up. I'd hoped that we could start this new journey together but she's not able or willing to look inwards it's too painful for her. It soon dawned on me that all we had was drinking and drugs, without that there was nothing, no common ground.

The things that I love most in my life are peace, tranquillity, calm, love and affection; she's the polar opposite of that. She's confrontational, aggressive, she swears, she's angry, she's racist, she's everything I'm not. When we started out, it was good fun and I could turn a blind eye to it all. I can no longer ignore all of the bits that I don't like. I hadn't been happy for years before but I didn't have the strength to leave. I felt this was what I deserved; I made my bed now I must lie in it. I was trapped, I thought my life was mapped out. It was only through recovery that I started to look after myself and to say this isn't healthy for me. I didn't want another broken family; it's having a negative effect on my children because they're not able to see the genuine me. My values were being trampled all over and subdued, so I took the decision that they would have a better version of me, not in that relationship.

I think that the children would have a more positive upbringing if they were with me but I'm not about to tear the family apart, so all I can hope for is that I can be as big a positive influence in their lives as I can be.

David's Story

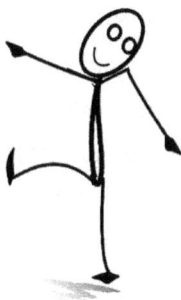

I'm an Anglican priest but retired. I've been retired a long time, since I was 37 when I had a colossal breakdown which took many years to recover. I was in an Anglican Parish here in County Durham when that happened. My upbringing was in the Church of England with parents who believed in God and went to church.

My father was a serving naval officer and fairly soon after I was born, he had to go to Malta to be captain of a ship in the British Fleet. My mother, my older brother and I lived there for a bit until he came back. That was his last ship and so he became a naval officer on dry land working at the admiralty and establishing a home in a leafy suburb of London, where a third brother was later born.

We went to private schools, which was important

163

to my parents and we boarded. I was the supposedly clever one of the family and times were relatively hard for my parents. A naval pension wasn't much and he retired compulsorily when he was 49, after 35 years in the Navy. I remember that funds were running out to support two of us and if I didn't get a scholarship to the public school, I'd have to go to grammar school. That, according to the family narrative, was a bit of a letdown. At least, that is what it felt like at the time. I had to take the '11 Plus' test as it was then, in the event I didn't win a scholarship to this public school but I did receive a scholarship.

By the time I was an adolescent, I had committed my life to Christ at a summer camp and I'd also started feeling this narrative of needing to succeed, needing to exceed, needing to obey, needing to do everything right.

That describes the start of my journey with depression. I found it very hard to be away from home and didn't like the public school, experience and education. I had a feeling more and more that I had to get on with it and produce. "Big Boys Don't Cry", was what my mother said to me when I was a youngster. When your mum tells you and you're a kid, you have to get on with it and perform but I'm crying and I don't need to tell you that. What I'm describing is a recipe for a collision course.

My commitment to Christ was a commitment deeper into another system of justification through works. I was in a church with an evangelical tradition but within the evangelical world of my youth 50 years ago there was a lot of law masquerading as Grace. That did not help me at all but at the age of 15, I felt the call to ordination. A Christian leader of the camps, in which I was converted, asked me what I wanted to do in life, and I said, "Well I want to go into the church," meaning ordination.

He corrected me and told me, "Oh, you're already in the church." I think the inference of my using that phrase was, that somehow ordained life was better than not being ordained. I was ordained 11 years later. I believe that sometimes God calls people to ordained ministry because he doesn't trust them as lay people and I can testify to that. Anyway, I went to University and Theological College, I met my wife and we were married six weeks after ordination. I served in a very lively strong Evangelical Church on Merseyside for four years and then moved to

Nottinghamshire to work with a wonderful man who served in Chile as a lay person and then was called to ministry. After that, I had my own parish in County Durham.

I was a raving charismatic back in those days and had been greatly impressed by The Fountain Trust, and people like Michael Harper, David Watson and others. We saw them as outstanding leaders and I guess part of me wanted to grab and copy what they seemed to be representing. I did have a real authentic experience of the Holy Spirit and liberation of much of my personality but there was also this deep seam of legalism and having to deliver, having to perform, having to succeed. The man who appointed me to my Parish wanted me to be an achiever, to deliver results in transforming the parish. A lot of the results of ministry there were good, and some were bad. There was a collision between spiritual life and spiritual darkness. A lot of people did come to Christ though and were filled with His spirit.

The church was growing but there was a backlash as well aimed personally at me and that was hard. I was also being treated for depression and I got M.E. which weakened me quite a bit. My thinking was that somehow God was going to bring me into greater freedom and liberty than I had at the time.

Then, in November 1987 I hit a brick wall, or I think of it as coming to hit me when I had a breakdown. I remember a dear lady coming to see me to offload her story about her family in my study. We were sitting opposite each other and she talked and talked and talked and I found myself receding into anxiety and a sense of losing connection with her. I was just feeling ill and that was the start of a spiral down into deep depression and anxiety.

Although we stayed living where we were, I was never well enough to go back into ministry and the church authorities gave me a full pension and support. We found a house for them to buy in Durham some miles away from the parish and they bought it. We lived there for a few years and all the time I was being treated with one drug therapy after another. That was well over 30 years ago and I have continued ever since to have cycles of wellness followed by a sudden spiral down into very severe depression and blackness; reaching a point where self-harm or suicide felt like a friend. Though I have never actually attempted anything the thoughts in your mind are very real and very distressing.

Near the start of this whole period, back in early 1988, I started to write poetry or rather it spilt out. I've been writing ever since. At first, it was just therapeutic, you know, cathartic. I tried to understand what was happening and to express it. I didn't have a pulpit to preach from, but I had poems to write to myself and others who cared to hear them. Although I knew that God was with me, this was really a hurting soul, a bit like, though not on the same level, the psalmists who often wrote a lament. Why are you so far from me? That sort of thing.

I found that as the poetry took up the shape of reflection on scripture and response to scripture, I was able to, in a way, give the depression, not a label but a shape. For instance, years before, I'd been given a wooden plaque from Africa carved by a depressed man, with words in Latin, De Profundis Clamavi. The translation reads, 'Out of the depths have I cried unto thee O Lord', which is from Psalm 130. I have it on a window ledge in my man cave.

I wrote a poem in which here I was in the depths,

in the pit crying out to God and it wasn't until He coughed, and I looked around that I thought, 'He's there.' You know, He was there in the depths, in the pit. I heard Him cough in a poem. I must have had that thought in my mind. I was so distracted but God was there to help me climb out. Quite a few years later in the middle of deep depression and winter, coming up to Christmas, the family was downstairs, I was upstairs. I was trying to work out how to end my life in the least hurtful way. I was on my bed, it was dark outside, there were no lights on in the room, it was very, very dark and then I saw out of my mind's eye a ragged shape on the wall. It was darker than the darkness within me, in the room and outside. I knew that's where Christ was, and that Christ had gone deeper into the darkness than I ever would and that was a fantastic 'WOW' moment and I put it into a poem in one of my books. This is what I wrote later, on 6th April 2001.

That Deeper Darkness

Birthed in an up-alley-café, amid generous,
kind, laughing, over-spilling hospitality,
who'd have known, imagined, suggested,
that this poem could actually have

been conceived in that deeper darkness,
that winter-never-ending blackness,
that Christmas-crushing, hope-smashing,
inner utter awfulness
that the un-ill-with-it may never realise
needs to be named, owned, capitalised,
there-I've-said-it Depression.

The light at the end of the tunnel
(so, say all of us Depressives
only a quarter joking)
is the train coming to smash you?

The deeper darkness,
that smear you only just see
out of the corner of your mind's eye
as you contemplate ending it all,
that not-so-much-no-go area as a
darkness-he's-gone-further-into-than-anyone-else,
is where Christ is.

© David Grieve
From my collection, 'Hope in Dark Places'
published by Sacristy Press, Durham. 2017
sacristy.co.uk

I've since come further, I now think that it wasn't
just Christ sharing my darkness and our darkness

but that we are sharing His; as part of the work, for me, of ministry and the vocation of a depressed Christian and depressed Theologian and poet, who can hand over to Christ and take on some of His sufferings. Saint Paul writes about somehow filling up the sufferings of Christ (Colossians 1:24, Philippians 3:10-11)

I see my calling, apart from the family calling, to be a priest and a poet and a depressive and I also say fidget because I have a magpie mind. That moment that I've described, where I saw Christ going deeper into the darkness than I'd been, has been formative over many years. It's formed the basis of the University of Life and the University of studying depression from the inside for many years.

This epiphany moment happened during the winter but it's not just a seasonal depression, it can happen at any time of the year and lasts on average three or four months. Usually, something good happens and I spring up again. The medication and the medical therapy have gone on and on and I was diagnosed as having Uni-Polar depression, the black without the elation for many years. Treatment-resistant depression was another diagnosis and generalized anxiety disorder.

Then a year ago we were having a post-Easter break on Holy Island (Lindisfarne) and I was terribly anxious and terribly depressed and I thought to myself, well the medication is not helping me, not that I can feel. I mean, there is a buffer zone element with every therapy that helps to stop you from killing yourself, but it wasn't making me well. I told my wife that I was going to ask for a fresh diagnosis and my doctor referred me back to the Mental Health Trust because I'd been signed off some years before. I had been well for three visits from a case worker. He signed me off and they drew up a plan to help me to stay well, which did not work.

So, I was referred back to the mental health forum for older people, the Wrinklies Department I call it. It was a different team from any I'd seen before and my psychiatrist diagnosed me as having Bipolar-Two. There are five different types of Bipolar and number two has the same plunges but not the same high elation and mania. So, I was put on an antipsychotic drug which is helpful. I've been on it for six months or more now and also have been having psychotherapy until recently. I've worked through a plan and learned about CAT therapy, which has nothing to do with felines. It is Cognitive Analytical Therapy. Rather than CBT, which is about behaviours, it's going right back into the areas that I talked about at the start of my story. It looks at the family and nurture and the hard-wiring, so we had a good look at that.

At the start of the therapy, I said I wanted to have more tools in the toolbox and to know how to use them. I wanted to understand this diagnosis and what it means. In my notebook, I wrote down the tools that I was using and my thinking and the poetry was flowering again. When I came out of illness this winter around the end of March, it started a whole spurt of theology in poetry and mindfulness and reflection and thanks and praise and so on.

I have this conviction that we're working with Christ, who we know is risen and glorified and yet with us still. We are experiencing some of what He experienced and experienced in a very real way. He suffered not just physically horribly but mentally horribly as well; this was a revelation to me.

I wrote a poem some years ago where I pictured

myself weeping, writing it at a time when I wasn't depressed. It was wintertime and I had had periods of weeping for other people, I knew it wasn't for myself but for other things. In the poem I was sitting down, probably on a step or something, weeping, and the Lord sat down beside me. He was also weeping and I felt very embarrassed about that. He said, "Just weep. Here's a bottle, cry into it, I know what tears are like." Then the poem switched to Gethsemane and Christ pouring out his heart with all those tears and again me being embarrassed because I couldn't get him to stop crying and I couldn't stop my own crying. That's a sense of the fellowship each individual can have with Christ the sufferer and the wounded healer. It is certainly a great comfort but also, it is reality and an inspiration to me.

I finished my therapy course but I'll be seeing the psychiatrist again next month. I have new mental concepts as part of the toolbox and a new assurance that things are going to be better. If I do begin to spiral down, I have ways to stop the hooks from getting in.

There is hope.

Martin's Story

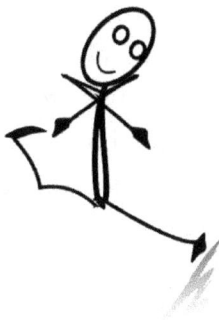

If we don't start talking about mental health it's never going to come out in the open, we can't talk enough about it because it just keeps getting pushed back. There's a battle between stigma and opening up. I think some men are their own worst enemies with it; we're not talking about this, it's unmanly rubbish. It is not unmanly to admit you're a human being and we're all human. I mean there are stories of people in the war soldiers who are crying over their dead buddy. Why is that unmanly? Somebody they've known for months and been under fire with and all sorts of things they've gone through, they get killed. They cry and that's shown in war films as well. So, why are we surprised when men do cry over things that are not necessarily as traumatic but still traumatic enough? If a man cries over his divorce, why are we putting him down? I know it's traumatic enough.

I've suffered different depressions my entire life, partly because I'm autistic and partly from some mental and emotional abuse from my mother and physical abuse from my brothers. Back in the 70s, you weren't autistic, you were just a pain in the backside. So, it has been hard and led to three suicide attempts in my life, depression and misery but I'm still alive and I have three lovely kids all in their 20s now.

My story starts in childhood. I've never felt part of anything except for a couple of years when I started attending church and I actually felt cared for then, but not understood. There was still that stigma around mental illness with many people but at least I was accepted, even if not understood. I met my now ex-wife through the church, but that didn't go well. I concluded a few years back, many years after the divorce, that people marry for the wrong reasons. They marry you for financial gain, for financial stability, instead of feeling like they can't live without that person.

I have things going through my head, little things I want to talk about, which you can only do with somebody who listens. They might not necessarily think the same way but they have time to listen without putting you down. That's another thing with men's mental health we can say these things that are in our minds, only to open ourselves up to condemnation, so the fear of that means we just don't bother.

I've noticed the way men communicate, we don't say much, we just sort of do head nods. We nod hello or get that and fine, it's a lot of body language. We can spend an hour in a pub, watching football with somebody for two hours and not even know their name, having a good time. When you get back home and the misses or the girlfriend says, "Did you have a good time?"

"Yeah."

"Who'd you meet?"

"Few blokes."

"What are their names?" They're amazed at that and how we can just watch football. Friendships for men are like that. We can sit there putting a piece of Lego together and have fun and not say a word. You can have some deep friendships that way, it depends on how you define deep, if it gives you comfort it's deep enough. I mean how many deep friends do you really need? You have casual acquaintances at work and then you've got friends that you'll just spend time with and other relationships like deeper friendships. You only need a few of those but if you haven't got that, that's where mental health issues can come up. As for me, I never had one at all but I'd rather be on my own and lonely than in a relationship and lonelier. I've been in both situations and I don't like being alone or lonely but it's preferable; I make decisions and don't get abused.

My mental health problems are basically the rhythm of my life. When I was younger, I thought it would get better the next year or it'll get better when I went to secondary school. It didn't, it got worse! I just tried to look forward to the next thing. It'll get better when I get out to work, it didn't and then my first suicide attempt came along just before my 18th birthday.

It was the early part of the year and we'd had a party via work because that's the only social life I had at the time. I realised how alone I was. I thought, 'I can't keep doing this.' I was making model kits at the time and I took a modelling knife, put it against my wrist and made a small cut – yikes! There's part of me that still winces now at the thought of it. It gave me a shock but was nothing more than a paper cut, so I just kept going on with life.

I worked for a bank for three years one month and 18 days and I hated it. One of the last things I did with that bank was go on a course and again I thought let's see what friends I can make. Once again, I was the outcast, I don't know why, I just was and I thought 'That's it,' so I took an overdose. I decided to stay at the hostel in Teddington at the bank's expense. I remember lying on the bed and listening to the song Mad World by Tears for Fears. The words of the song were, '*The dreams in which I'm dying are the best I've ever had.*' It's peculiar when you get to that point, it is the most content you've been because you think it's ending now. I don't know if they find suicidal people who've killed themselves with a smile on their faces. If they do, that's probably why.

Anyway, back to what is a weird story. Every time I think about it, it gets weirder. It was the last night of this course and people were getting drunk and I was having a few drinks with the group. It wasn't going well, I felt left out even more, so I went to the room and started taking aspirin. These were the days when you could buy 200 aspirin in a big bottle. Of course, the pharmacist looked at me. I said, I just want to keep them at home. I'm dressed in a suit, I look normal, so he put them in a bag. Then I went to the off-license, bought a load of bottles of cider, smuggled them back into the hostel and thought, 'I'm gonna give this one last chance again.' I went downstairs and they were still winding me up. I thought 'screw it', so went upstairs and started drinking and popping the pills, feeling happy and then, one of the girls on the course came into the room. She invited me to a party upstairs in her room. I thought, 'You know what the hell, I can finish killing myself later.' I went upstairs and while I sobered up, I thought nah, I'm not gonna do this. Did I have a headache the following morning! I think I got through 50 soluble aspirin that night. How the hell I still had a headache the following morning I don't know but I did not feel well, so that's how it ended. There were just two years between my first and second suicide attempts when I was age 20. During those two years, life hadn't really gotten any better and I thought screw this, the job was horrible.

Getting bullied at work by an assistant manager as well, didn't help. Rod got his comeuppance later on because after this I thought screw this I'm going on holiday. He said, "No you can't go because we've got two people off, it will be too many people off in that department."

I thought screw this, I've already handed my notice in. I just went and after a week the branch manager called me up at home and of course, I wasn't there because I decided to stay on holiday for a second week. I thought screw it, what are they gonna do, fire me? That's when my mum stepped in, one of the few occasions she did stand up for me. She was odd in some ways. She did have a love for me but it was tempered with a desire to control and domineer. We saw a psychiatrist when I was eight but I didn't know she was seeing one at the same time apparently. I was silently rebellious and I just refused to open up. They told her she was domineering, she disagreed with it and that's the last time we went. I was 38 when she said this. I just looked at her and thought I'm not saying a word here Mother because you are, you were and you always will be. She still was even to her dying day so, yeah, I had that growing up all the time.

I left the bank and went to work in the pub over the road, it was one of the best things I ever did. I was approaching my 21st birthday and I thought, 'What is the point of all this? What is the real point? That's when I came across Christianity for the first time and I thought, 'Okay this gives me something.' I think God was reaching into my life at that point and saying, 'Okay it's been rough let's get you on a slightly different path.'

I worked through it but there were ups and downs. I thought what if I die now, I'll get to meet God? I came to this independently, I don't regret it at all, I don't go to a church at the moment because I tend to have disagreements with doctrine. I still maintain my faith and while I'm looking forward to what comes next, I'm not in a hurry to get there

All those experiences when I was young made me a more compassionate person, often to the point of detriment of my own health, just to feel useful. When you need to feel accepted, you will forgive a whole load of rubbish that you shouldn't. You will help people who hurt you. It takes a lot to give yourself some backbone because everyone needs to be accepted. We do it with kids when they're very young, you know, oh you pooped in your pants, don't worry you just wipe it up, it happens. We'll do that sort of thing because they're kids and as they get older, we change to an extent and we don't accept them enough.

My eldest is also autistic, his mother was really good and had him diagnosed but she tried to change him. I just take him as he is and he's probably a decade behind in some regards but he's got a better sense of himself than I ever had. He doesn't need acceptance from other people because he gets acceptance from me and if he wants to chat and unload, he always makes sure I'm ready for it. Then, when we do chat, I've been able to use that part of my life to help him and to help others as well. I always wanted kids anyway but they give me that purpose. It does make life easier but it's still not easy because although that's a purpose, it's not an acceptance of who you are. In I.T. terms it's a workaround, not a fix, it doesn't fix the initial problem which is lack of acceptance.

I've had lots of low moments, times I cried and times that I wanted to. I've been on antidepressants for most of the last 14 years. I'll be coming off them this year because I've got some other support now. Up until this year, I didn't really feel I had any support, then I had suicidal thoughts after some nasty shenanigans at work but instead of reaching for pills or anything like that, I reached for a phone and called a helpline and after 20 minutes into the call, I thought I feel better just for letting it out. I now know that I don't need the pills when I've got that backup, so that's a step forward.

My third suicide attempt happened just after I was divorced in 2007. We still shared the house for another two years [till 2009] and I slept on the sofa. Then after that, she manipulated her way to a council house. I don't know what she was telling her lawyer and other people but I was certainly made out to be the bad guy, even though she's the one who had the affair and I divorced her because of it.

I ended up with nothing. We had the joint account which was nearly empty. I had no income because I was unemployed. She got a house, the kids, everything and so I made another plan. I got a bottle of white wine and I'd spent several days getting Nurofen from various places. By then, I was staying at my mum's and she was giving me grief as well. Why aren't you out getting a job? I had just gone through a divorce and I was dazed and confused, I didn't know what was happening. There was no sympathy there at all.

I remember watching Vanilla Sky on the Telly with Tom Cruise, not a bad film actually, drinking away and just taking the pills and then falling asleep thinking this is it it's all over. I woke up the following morning. My mum is standing over me, seeing all the pill packets on the floor and the empty bottle of wine. All I did was look at her and say, "Why am I still alive?"

I think it was the biggest shock to her system she'd ever had. She mellowed a lot after that but it took that much. I went to the hospital for several blood tests and eventually, a counsellor came in and decided to refer me to the mental health services. I started seeing a counsellor and social worker after that.

It's been up and down since then and it's taken a long time. I've had problems with neighbours and problems at work, problems here, there and everywherc. A few months later, my eldest moved in with me at my mum's place because now my ex-wife had the house, she wanted to make sure she had it to herself. She slowly worked it out that way and one after the other, all three of my kids left. Two of them live with me in the flat at the moment.

I'm getting therapy as well at the moment. I've been doing it for a few weeks. Now I think I'm not in a hurry to die, death comes when it comes. It will come to us all at some point, it's a question of when. I mean, I'm 60 now, so I've effectively two more decades left before I will die. If I live longer, I live longer. If I don't live as long, it is what it is. I mean I'm in the last part of my life and when I talk to the younger people that I work with about this, they can't cope with it. They're all around 30ish, I just call them kids as part of the banter. They can't quite get their heads around what I say. I notice as well now that there's a lot of banter at work about my age but they appreciate the life experience I have. So, I know I'm useful in some way but it's not that deep personal acceptance that everyone needs. I may never get that. Though I feel valued now a little more than I did, there's still that anxiety thinking. Most days I think that they're going to fire me but it never happens.

Another thing I found out over the last decade or so is about forgiveness. It was pointed out to me that it's not about the other person, forgiveness is so you can move on, even if they are still horrible. It doesn't change them it changes you. That was something I never had before. It took me years to realise that forgiveness is not about the other person, it's to enable you to move on without bitterness, which came as a shock and surprise and pleasant.

Look, how do you forgive somebody who's hurt you that badly? You don't, you just stop them from dominating your life and it takes time to do that. You can't easily do it. My ex is still as manipulative as ever, I've barely spoken to her in 14 years but the things she does and says, I mean my eldest doesn't trust her. She kicked my youngest out when they disagreed and he spent a summer night on a park bench. Then I helped him to get into another flat and he's now shacked up with his girlfriend. He's settled and keeps in touch now. His girlfriend will make sure he keeps ringing me, she's got her feet solidly on the ground. I try to be a good dad to my kids and do fun things with them. I still have bad moments and don't like mornings, I'm grumpy as hell in the morning. When I leave for work, I try to put on this face to the outside world.

Talking about suicides and depression and things is not something I do unless people are interested or want to know. I feel that's like a lot of comedians from the past they try and make life better for others, better than they have. Robin Williams and Tony Hancock were great examples of that. I admire people like that but sadly, they both took their own lives because I don't think they ever really got the attention that everyone needs. They were seen as stars rather than anything else and I'm sure there are lots of other famous people over the years who've done the same. There will also be tens of thousands of non-famous people who did that and they just ran out of energy one day.

I've given a lot of thought to mental health and suicide and things. I've concluded there are only two reasons people kill themselves; they've run out of reasons to live or they want to die. These are two separate things. For the first, if you give them another reason to live, they'll go on. The second lot is much harder to help. We seem to have this obsession with keeping people alive without changing their situation. Unless you change the reason why they feel the way they do, aren't they just going to go back and do it again? I wonder if it's because the people trying to stop them don't want to be reminded that other people do not have a good time. I wonder if that's what's behind this covering up of men's Mental Health. The thought of, I don't want to face this therefore I'm shutting him up, I don't want to be exposed to a hole in my life, so I'm shutting them up, I'm not having that anymore.

Anyone who tries to put down men's mental health gets a fairly stern answer from me these days. I don't let them run with it. Look at Gary Speed the Welsh footballer and manager, who killed himself and that brought on a lot of discussion about mental health. I even heard somebody stupidly say that he took the coward's way out. No, cowards don't kill themselves, cowards run away from their problems, brave people face them and sometimes you're just not brave enough. It's easy to be brave when you're in a group and so much more difficult when on your own. If you're on your own, bravery will expire. It's like love in a way. It's bottomless you can run out of it by yourself, yet when you're with somebody who cares, you both charge each other up.

With bravery sometimes you just need a squeeze of the hand or a hug and you can go through the rest of the day or the rest of the week it doesn't take a lot to charge. It's like a five-minute charge of an electric bike for instance. I think we've so many analogies we can use these days that weren't there in the past. Maybe it's like eating a slice of bread that just satisfies the hunger, it doesn't take much.

It is so important to talk out when you're feeling low. Though for some people it's not easy if you were brought up to hide everything. It's one of the most difficult things you will ever have to do and it takes a complete change of thinking before you can. When I called the helpline, I'd slowly got used to opening up and of course, these people, you'll never bump into them. They're not even recorded and you can just open up to them knowing that you're not going to get judged. They're not going to put you down, they won't give you advice but often you don't need that, you just need to talk it out. Then you will be able to say, I know what I need to do.

It's useful trying to change those habits but trying to change those methods of thinking is very difficult and, in some cases, very painful, especially if there's a lack of trust. When you get to that point of loneliness you have a lack of trust in other people and other things, so it is a big difficulty, especially for men. I think it's worse if you've been brought up in a manly way because you hide it or you drink or you get drugs and you just deal with it that way. One of my favourite historical stories is from the Vietnam War. Half of the soldiers were high on Heroin half the time and Americans feared they were going to have a massive drug problem when they came back to the States. It never materialised because they were then in a new situation and they didn't have the problems associated with the Vietnam War, so you change the situation and you do not necessarily get the same problems. If we open up this idea about getting men to talk, a lot of problems will disappear but there will still be the ones we need to deal with, sadness and loneliness are always going to be there. It's a question of how we help people deal with it.

Doc's story

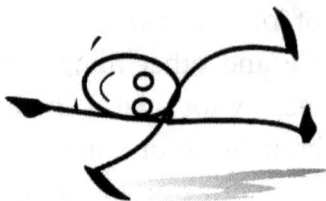

In 1991 I was playing softball for an organisation and I was running to home plate. It's a friendly game, the catcher and I bumped shoulders and I went flying off of him. I hit a metal pole with my head. I fractured my skull and my eye came out of my head and I stopped breathing twice on the field. The ambulance people got me breathing and took me to the hospital. I have eight plates and 32 screws in my head and it took me forever to recover. I have a problem talking, sleeping, walking and everything else that you can imagine that takes play in someone's day. That's what we tend to say was the starting point of the depression. The doctors said that the accident could have triggered it.

From that point on it's been a very crazy road. I was presenting a cable TV show called 'Wrestling Tracks USA' and it was on every week. I was one of the crazy guys from wrestling who came out and dressed like one of those fools that you see every week on television yelling and screaming. It was a lot of fun. A police department saw the show and they had a phenomenal video production team, they asked if I would be interested in doing a show together called, 'Body Slam on Drugs', it was an anti-drug show, so I agreed.

Every week, I would come out in the studio in my red white and blue outfit. I'd be yelling and screaming like a madman; we'd have guests on and we'd even show a wrestling clip. It was all geared towards the kids, to help them stay away from drugs. After three years the show ended and the police officer and I decided to do a radio show and we called it 'Outlaws for Christ Radio.'

It was a Christian-based radio show which ran for three years and then I did another show called, 'Outlaw and the Blue' a blues music show. At that point, for the most of 15 years since my accident, I was sick the whole time with depression. There was one point when we were in a studio and we were recording five shows in one night. I was still doing the cable TV show and I was struggling to do it. Looking back at it now, I can't believe how much I was struggling. We were just finishing up the show and I turned around and said to everybody, "This is my last show, I can't do this anymore."

I turned around and I walked out of the studio. I went home and was miserable for months. I became suicidal and it was so strong. I also worked for a bus company for 30 years helping disabled children. Everybody knew something was wrong with me but only one of them said anything. A black girl who was young enough to be my daughter came up and said, "I know something's wrong with you."

Every day she would sit by me in the morning and after work; she would sit and talk with me every day. One day we sat on a wooden bench against a building and she said to me, "Most nights when I pray, I fall asleep during prayer. Last night I sat up and prayed and asked the Lord to protect you, bless you and be by your side."

The way that she said it really hit me but I kept spiralling out of control. I reached the point where I almost died from an overdose of pills. They took me to the hospital where I spent seven or eight days; that was the first time that I was there. I wanted to die but I didn't have the nerve to kill myself you know it's a crazy thing. I wish you could be in my head, so you could understand what I'm saying because even in the hospital it was such a crazy thing. People were coming up and talking to me asking what they should do. I would say, "You know I'm a patient, right?"

At one point the nurses went up to my wife and they said I should be a counsellor because I was counselling more people in the hospital than they were. On my first hospital visit, I stayed in the emergency room for the weekend. For some reason, they had a rule that they couldn't bring you into the psychiatric area until Monday morning.

There was me and three other guys and one guy attempted suicide. He took a gun, pointed it at his head and he fired, but it misfired. He had a ring on his head, there was smoke and a burn. Another guy was an alcoholic, he fell and busted up his face and then another guy was paralyzed and they were all talking to me. My wife wondered why they were all coming to me, as we were all there for the same reason. On Saturday morning, the day after I was admitted, my wife brought in chicken cutlets, enough for everyone.

So, I'm sitting on this bed and I'm saying to these other guys, "Who wants some chicken?"

They all tasted it and the guy that tried to kill himself said, "Wow this is so good."

I said to him, "I want to tell you something, if your gun had not misfired, you wouldn't be eating this chicken."

He looked at me and said, "You know you're right." It's like I was supposed to be there but for another reason.

At times, the hospital staff treats the patients like children, especially around snack time. It was during one of these snack times that I met another black girl standing in front of me. I looked down and noticed on her right arm she had a tattoo of Jesus upside down. I said to her, "That tattoo is very interesting." She responded by calmly telling me that He is her brother.

We sat down together and started talking. Well, she was talking. She would look to her left or right and act like she was talking to somebody who wasn't there. We talked a lot and she told me about brother Jesus. On the day I was leaving, I was in a hallway and she was there in a white gown. I told her I was leaving and she told me that she was sorry to see me go. She reached her arms out in my direction and as I was walking over to her to say goodbye, my daughter asked me what was going on and I said jokingly, "Hey that's Jesus's sister and now I have a connection to Him."

I walked to the girl and when I hugged her goodbye, it was like electricity came out of her hands, it just felt like my whole body was vibrant. I was just totally stunned, now all these years have gone by I think of that almost every day. It impacted me so much.

Another strange thing happened whilst I was in the hospital, an American Native Indian doctor suggested that I should write poetry. At that time, I thought he was crazier than me and I said just leave me alone I'm not going to write but he insisted and gave me a pad of paper and a pencil. He shut me into a room by myself, closed the door and said, "Start writing I'll be back in an hour."

I wrote a poem called, 'That's the beauty of it all' and I have no idea where that came from. I looked at it and was totally stunned. Even the doctor was shocked when he came back. It wasn't a great poem but it made sense. He asked where it came from. I told him I had no idea. I thought to myself, they wouldn't tell a guy who's in a mental hospital that his poem was terrible, that might just push him over the edge. Then, he asked me to write another poem and I wrote one about that black girl I was telling you about, I called it, 'When God's angel became my friend.'

I wrote a third poem called, 'Lord did you forget about me?' The hospital staff and my wife struggled to believe that I had written the poems. I've been writing ever since.

In 2021 I became very ill physically. It was triggered by catching Covid, then having a Covid vaccination and I then became ill again. I didn't get better and it got worse and worse and worse. They called it 'Long Haulers syndrome (Long Covid in the UK). It was just horrible, to the point that I thought I would never recover. Eventually, I was diagnosed with 'Lambert Eaton Syndrome', it's like a cousin of muscular dystrophy.

My walking has become more difficult, I have

less energy and I can lose my voice in an instant. It comes back a half hour or two days later. It can be depressing. I would no longer consider suicide as an option but the depression does hit a lot. I have two different types of dark days, one is with full-on depression, I mean it's just like being in a giant hole that you can't get out of. Then, there are days with no hope and you feel trapped.

I learned a little trick and that helps me. I tell myself to forget about this for now and go lay down, forget about it, it'll be okay tomorrow and it works a lot. There are dark days when I don't want to talk to anybody, I don't want to be around anybody. If I could sit in a darkened room and close the door and nobody came in, I would be okay with that. I would still be miserable. In fact, I'll take it a step further, if there was a box in the room that I could crawl into, that would be even better. I'm pretty open about it, I just don't want to see anyone. I talk about it because I've belonged to a mental health association for years; I've done some talks for them and I try to inject some humour into it. We all need that.

I'm being honest with you when I say, I believe my strength comes from Jesus and God. I want to be better than I am but I struggle. I remember when I was in the hospital, especially the last time and I was writing all these poems. They were coming very easy and everything talked about God and Jesus, an angel and heaven. This was God's gift to me. I'm such a big believer in God's gifts that it just drives me crazy when other people can't see it, I mean I want to grab them and shake them.

When I was in the hospital, I decided that I wanted to get baptised. I don't have a clue how I thought that. So, when I got out of the hospital, I started going to this church and after three or four months, they're going to have a baptism. Now, I was already baptised when I was a kid but I wanted it that much I said to the pastor, "I'm really interested, in fact, I absolutely want this."

I didn't tell my family I didn't tell anyone. Then, a few days before I was being baptised, I asked my wife and my daughter to come to church with me on Sunday. They both agreed and you should have seen the look on their faces when I got up and was baptised. Some years later I decided to be ordained through the National Association of Christian Ministers I felt like I needed to do it for me but it has provided me with more purpose and I actually ended up being asked to officiate at eleven weddings and I never charged a dime, I just couldn't. To me, it was a God thing and there was no charge for that.

I live with depression and bipolar and it can be a struggle to stay on the right path. Your world can be unsettling, to say the least. For me, it's given me time to think and come to the conclusion that mental illness is like an epidemic. Suicide in the States is skyrocketing for not only the youth but for every age group and it does not seem like it is slowing down at all. They could never imagine in all their days that they would witness the things that they are seeing now, and people are worried about the fake news and lies that they hear.

One of the ways that I cope with life is to spend a lot of time sitting outside in a tiny porch-like area that I call my place of grace. I even eat most of my meals there and I am more in tune with nature and my surroundings. While listening to the radio and television I started to realise people were intent on hurting each other for causes they did not even understand. Many folks were becoming disrespectful and flat-out rude while others who were trying to tell their own stories were being told to shut up or even threatened. I started listening and reading about these different events and that is when I wrote this poem.

TO THOSE

⊙ Oct 13, 2021 - The Depressed Poet, Doc Dalton

Give love to those who live without it
Bring friendship to those who are lonely
Give hope to those who are hopeless
Bring peace to the hearts of those who are weary
Show faith to those who are in search of it
Give honesty to those who have been lied to
Share your wisdom with those who have suffered
from life's lessons
Show understanding to those who are in doubt
Find a path for those who are lost and
cannot find their way
Bring light for those depressed and
live in the shadows of darkness
Give strength to those who struggle
and have weakened
Bring a smile to those faces who
wear their sadness
Explain to those who are truly
in search of answers
Listen to those who need to have
their stories told

202

Pray for those who need your prayers the most
Together let's pray to the Father, Son, and Holy
Ghost

Here's a thing about mental health, there are times when people might look at you or judge you. This could hurt you big time because instead of focusing on yourself to become a better you, you are now focusing on a place that does nothing for you. You try to please them, people who you don't even know. What you need to do is change your so-called direction and get back to what is important and that is you and your personal wellbeing.

For me, it is simple and straight to the point. I don't give a rat's ass what anyone thinks. That is on them. You must have a big pair of balls to look down on someone who is struggling. This makes them a person who needs to find their own peace and happiness within their own, hell hole of a life.

This so-called mental health journey can be a long and lonely one, even when that journey takes place in your mind while never leaving the comfort of your favourite chair. The journey can change within your mind at any given time and can take you on a different path even if you do not want to go on one. The places that you go to and come from in your mind can be exhausting and can challenge you in several ways. It can also be rewarding and bring you peace, something that you really need and deserve. As crazy as this might sound, there are moments when you say to yourself, I think this is the time to shut this journey down and to speak to someone.

If I had the power to change the world, I would want to see more kindness. We have become a people who are no longer kind to one another. Just how difficult is it to say good morning to someone or have a nice day? How tough is it to open a door for someone or maybe carry something that is difficult for someone to carry themselves? How hard is it to smile at someone or pat them on the back and tell them all will be, OK? Maybe just one act of kindness can help someone through their day. Maybe one act of kindness can go much farther than you could have ever imagined. If we behaved more like this, I believe that the world would be a better place and fewer people would struggle with their mental health.

Mike's Story

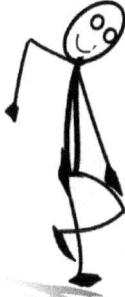

I was preaching the other day about Ephesians 2 verses 1 to 10. It describes our condition, and then in the middle, it says BUT God. I think, for anybody suffering a mental health issue that we come to that realisation, but God, we are this… but God.

Ephesians 2:1-10

And you He made alive, who were dead in trespasses and sins, [2] in which you once walked according to the [a] course of this world, according to the prince of the power of the air, the spirit who now works in the sons of disobedience, [3] among whom also we all once conducted ourselves in the lusts of our flesh, fulfilling the desires of the flesh and the mind, and were by nature children of wrath, just as the others.

*[4](#) **But God**, who is rich in mercy, because of His great love with which He loved us, [5] even when we were dead in trespasses, made us alive together with Christ (by grace you have been saved), [6] and raised us up together, and made us sit together in the heavenly places in Christ Jesus, [7] that in the ages to come He might show the exceeding riches of His grace in His kindness toward us in Christ Jesus. [8] For by grace you have been saved through faith, and that not of yourselves; it is the gift of God, [9] not of works, lest anyone should boast. [10] For we are His workmanship, created in Christ Jesus for good works, which God prepared beforehand that we should walk in them.*

I was born the youngest child of a family of five kids with me and Mum and Dad. Dad was not nice he was difficult to deal with. There were moments of absolute 'dadness' when he was a good dad. There were other times when it was horrendous. I suppose he had never been taught how to bring children up, he didn't know the first thing about what he was doing and after his time in the Army, I think he struggled. He was on the bulldozers that dealt with Belsen. You know the stories that we've heard and the things that we know about only touch the surface of what the guys had to deal with. They were 20 minutes on a bulldozer followed by a 2-hour break. It must have been awful and I think any trauma like that, has to turn a man. Some coped, some gave up completely and some like my dad, really struggled.

I know he wasn't a Christian most of his life and I didn't have that much Christian input until I was seven and then I started going to church. Also, at school, my headmaster was awful, he was worse than my dad in some ways. He would cane us for the little things. I remember once getting caned for watching a fight outside school, not during school hours, just because he thought it was wrong. So, I went through all that and lots of power struggles within the family and I started drinking. I started smoking when I was about 13 and I started drinking probably two or 3 weeks later, when I found that drinking dulled the pain and the thoughts. I didn't have to think about stuff and I didn't have to deal with interpersonal relationships, which I'd always found difficult. By the time I left school, I was drinking a lot. I was drinking spirits every day and then I got my driving license and I didn't drink so much because you don't drink and drive.

What else happened when I was 13? I was sexually abused and to this day I can't remember who it was. I know that it was somebody close and that they were male and it confused me sexually as well. Then, on top of all the other things, I went through a really rough patch when my dad died. I was 18, had just gotten my driving license and it was a difficult time watching him die. He was seriously ill for four or five years, so it was a slow painful death. They kept giving him experimental treatments to prolong his life, but by the time we reached the third or fourth treatment, I thought why bother? I know that is a horrible thing to say. My mum was nursing him all the time and struggling with everything she went through but that's another story.

I was the only child left at home by this time, so I was dealing with all of that and then, my sister got divorced. She had kids and lived just down the road, all those dynamics that were going on. Then, at the age of 20, I was married for the first time. It was not a good marriage, she had real mental issues and convinced me that my mental issues were worse than hers. I was doing all sorts of things and because I was naïve, needy and vulnerable in myself, I believed a lot of the lies. At one point I started to see a psychiatrist but eventually, after nine years, she decided to kick me out and divorce me. It was a nasty divorce and that sent me into a real tailspin.

I started going to a church locally but they were quite controlling. I suppose in some ways that was good for me at that time, as I was not in a good place. I did something wrong, something I shouldn't have done and I admit that freely but then they told me that God wanted nothing else to do with me because of what I'd done. Reading the Bible further on down the road and learning from some other men, I realised that they were wrong. At that time, it was the only thing that had kept me going at all and it had been taken away. I felt awful, I was just an empty shell and I started drinking more; a lot more. I began to lose myself in writing poetry, some of the darkest poetry I've ever written. I read some recently and it's really dark due to the difficult headspace that I was in. I could see no way out. The drink dulled it for a while and then it didn't.

People would say things to me, I'd get a bit upset and try to kill myself. I took so many overdoses and ended up in hospital so many times. I tried to hang myself but the rope stretched and my feet touched the ground. As that wasn't very successful, I tried to cut my wrist and went off and wandered around the streets for a bit, trying to keep the blood pumping so I could bleed out. The police arrested me and I was sectioned and taken to the local psychiatric hospital but they weren't really bothered. They just wanted to drug me up, shove me in a corner and they eventually let me out after a week or two because I didn't want to talk to any of them. There was no diagnosis, absolutely nothing and so they kicked me out.

By this time my mum decided she couldn't have me back in the house, which is understandable, you don't want somebody who might try to kill themselves living with you when you're old and infirm. I had nowhere to go and I found a little bedsit and stayed there for a few years. While I was there, I started drinking a lot more than I had been. I was now drinking a litre of whiskey every day and topping it up with cheap wine, just to switch things off. I started smoking Cannabis and was taking prescription drugs, painkillers, anti-depressants and some other things that I can't remember. I was doing all that, all day every day. I woke up in the hospital so many times, after I had been found unconscious, passed out on the side of the road. Somebody would take me into hospital and I'd wake up the next morning and sign myself out and go and get another bottle of whiskey.

As boys, we were told that men don't cry, we're always told that and so you keep all the emotions in, particularly if you're a sexual abuse victim. You don't talk about those things, that can't happen to you because you're not a girl. All that builds up inside and then of course it's bothering you. You're struggling and people tell you that you're a bad person because of this or that and the other. It just goes on and on and on, it builds up and up and up and the only outlet you feel you have at that time is to have something that causes hurt. The hurt shows because there's no other way of doing it, no other and that was where I was. I was hurting myself and doing things like fighting with a lamppost. I remember one night I was drunk whilst walking down the middle of the road asking all the drivers that went past to run me over. I told them I wouldn't press charges either because I'd be dead.

I was arrested that night for assaulting a police officer because he surprised me from behind. My automatic reaction was to turn around and thump or kick in this case. This was the darkest time of my life. Then, as I said earlier, **'but God.'**

Somebody came around to the house where I was staying from the local church bringing Christian music CDs around for people to listen to. I was in the choir when I was a boy and right up until I was 18 years old and was always interested in Christian music. At that point in my life, I looked a little bit different to what I do now. I was certainly slimmer than I am now and had a kind of a wide Mohican haircut. It was bleached white with a blood-red point and I used to wear a leather jacket with drips of blood painted on the back. I had earrings and I looked horrible and grumpy and everything else to keep people away, like a defensive barrier.

I wouldn't go out of the house, if I had to go out it was always by the back streets. I didn't want to know anybody, speak to anybody, didn't want anything. I listened to music all the time as loud as I could, just to drown out and stop the thoughts in my mind. So, when he brought me this CD of Christian music, I sat down and listened to it at full volume through the headphones and it was loud. A version of the 23rd Psalm came on with an additional chorus, it's by Stuart Townend. The chorus says, 'I will trust in you alone.' Those words were playing and I kind of had a picture in my mind not quite a vision, not that sort of three-dimensional reality but I had a picture on my mind of somebody standing at the other end of the room in traditional Bible clothes. His arms were outstretched and He said, "Come home."

The emotion was so powerful that I literally ran across the room with my headphones flying one way and I tripped over the sofa. I ended up at the other side of the room just sobbing. This led me to start going to the church, not for their services at first. They were doing some singing as a choir, so I went to that and then I started going to the church. Shortly after that, I heard this voice in my head saying, "I want you to give it up."

It was so distinct from all the voices that were there accusing me of this and that. This was a still small voice. I wasn't quite sure what He wanted me to give up so I stopped everything apart from the tobacco. I stopped drinking, the drugs, the prescription stuff everything all at the same time and did it cold turkey for two or three days. That was it, I was still smoking but the rest had gone and you know that looking back and talking to other guys who've had issues with those substances that's a miracle.

That was my conversion if you like, the time I actually said, right I'm going to get serious about God and I'm going to believe in God and I trust in Him. I bumbled on at that level for several years and then eventually went back to live with my mum and started to work as a gardener. I was engaged to somebody else at the time but she was going off into all sorts of witchcraft and I wanted no part of it. Then I met my wife, the nice one and we just formed a relationship. At first, we met as friends and we would read and study the Bible together.

Fast forward a couple of years and I decided that I wouldn't be able to continue gardening commercially. That was when I thought it was time to start looking around for something else. I thought it would be nice to have a little tea shop in the Cotswolds, where we could just do what we like more or less and charge people for it, which is I suppose the Englishman's dream. I shared this with my wife for a few months, and then one morning I woke up and said, "I think God wants us to have Christian books in our Café."

She said, "I think you're right; I've been thinking

the same thing, I just didn't say it." I was still smoking tobacco at the time and I packed that up with some help and I started to buy books for the bookshop from the proceeds of not smoking. We ended up very quickly with a large quantity of books that we needed to shift. That was when we started going out and doing book selling around the local churches and events; until 2016 when we opened a shop.

About 3 years in perhaps, I can't remember the exact dates, things were at the point where they were so bad that I was planning to kill myself. It was just so bad and it was just after my daughter had been born. I planned it to the last detail, the time and everything, so that I wouldn't be discovered by my wife, I'd be discovered by the cleaners; they could clean it up. People kept saying to me at that time that I had so much to live for, and that my life was so good, but they didn't know what I was contemplating.

When your kids are little, people say things like that but I felt that the world would be better off without me. My wife and daughter would be better off without me, it's a hard place to be. I mean, if anybody hasn't been there you can't imagine how bad it is to be there. No amount of explaining can really tell you. I hope nobody reading this would ever come to that point.

I was about to go outside to end it and the phone rang. Now, I've got ADHD and I can't walk past a ringing phone without answering it; I just had to answer the phone. There was this guy, I knew him, he was one of the sales reps who phoned me every couple of weeks to talk about their new products and he said, "Mike, I'm sitting outside my office. I haven't gone into work yet as I just felt God tell me to phone you to pray with you."

He was in Eastbourne and I'm in Gloucestershire, 170 miles away. He had no way of knowing what was going on. He phoned me and prayed with me and it's hard to describe what that means to me now. Whatever our situation, whoever we are, if we belong to The Lord, we are right there in the palm of his hand. Even though we might think He's let go and dropped the ball. He's right there, able to save to the uttermost and that is incredible. It's incredible that God told a faithful man to make a phone call.

I didn't tell him then about what he had stopped me from doing but I did tell him when we met.

He saved my life with that call and it's an amazing thing. I still get bouts of depression but I remember that I'm in the palm of His hand. When I am depressed, I remember that; I turn to the Bible looking for words to come and I pray. I sometimes go into a dark room and scream and I'm not afraid to cry. Sometimes I'll phone somebody up or God has His way of sending somebody alongside.

I am a lot more aware of my mental health these days I suppose. Now I say, your feelings lie to you. There is a truth that is far greater than your feelings and that is what you have to cling to. Your feelings lie to you all the time, they say that you're worthless but you're not you have worth. You have so much worth that God sent His only Son for you, so that's how much you're worth, so you don't need to go to those dark places.

Find out more about Mike's shop at www.scrolleaters.com

Wrong for men

As I look back on my life
To the time when I was ten
As I began to grow up

In a world of big strong men
There was gravel in my gut
My arms were growing strong
My fists were bruised and bloody
But inside something was wrong
Deep inside this tough young boy
Was a loving tender side
And every time I loved and failed
My heart was broken wide

Tell me why, tell me why
Is it wrong for men to cry?

As I think back over years
That quickly passed me by
And I think of all the things I've lost
A tear wets my eye
But something stops it falling
And running down my face
Some little voice tells me
To cry is a disgrace
I'm tired of losing everything
I'm broken deep inside
I'm not sure if I can hold it in
But like the man I am, I'll try

Tell me why, tell me why
Is it wrong for men to cry?

I take the things that happen
And I bottle them inside
I try to forget the hurt
I felt when her love died
I try to forget the feelings
Of being hurt again
I try to laugh and joke and swear
Like other big strong men
But deep inside's a feeling
That I can't much longer hide
That everything would be better
If just for once I cried

Tell me why, tell me why
Is it wrong for men to cry?

I will die, I will die
Unless for once I cry

Tell me now, if I cry
Will man's strong image die

Tell me why, tell me why
Is it wrong for men to cry?

© *Michael S Juggins 2023*

Brian's Story

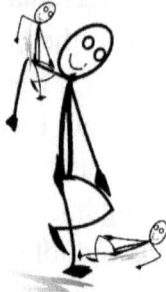

I was born in London in 1954 and two years later, we moved to Canvey Island, at the mouth of the river Thames. This is where I grew up with my father, who was a grocer, my mother who was a housewife and my younger sister Janice, born in 1957. Canvey Island was rural and I enjoyed nature and living in the countryside though I didn't care much for school. My favourite hobby was making plastic models.

I was a Boy Scout, and as I got older, I joined the Air Training Corp, a youth organisation run by the Royal Air Force. I naturally developed an interest in military matters. My father had taken part in the invasion of France (D-day) and several of my uncles also fought in the war. I was proud of my family and my heritage, so joined the army when I was 16 years old, as an army apprentice in the Royal Engineers. I studied military affairs, as well as the management of heavy equipment, excavators, bulldozers, etc.

I enjoyed military life, but it was then that I also started drinking a lot. It's almost endemic in the army, everybody does it. I remember one time when we had a weekend in the barracks and we just went to the NAAFI and bought crates and crates of beer and just spent the whole weekend drinking; we reached the point where we couldn't stand up and were sick as a dog. Sadly, when I went home, I was the same and I think I lost a lot of my friends because of my drinking. I'd go to parties and drink myself under the table; it was absolutely crazy. I never once considered myself an alcoholic, as I was just the same as everyone else.

I was promoted to corporal and served 7 years in the army before I left in 1977 and joined the police. It was then that it struck me that I couldn't carry on with the binge drinking and I started to calm down. I met my first wife during this time, she was also a police officer and our son was born in 1980, followed by our daughter three years later. I worked as a community police officer on a council estate in Chelmsford, Essex and the work started to upset me. I became discouraged and depressed.

I seemed to go from one petty crime to another; violence and neighbourhood disputes dragged me down. There was a positive side to the work as well; I used to go around schools and give educational talks, but I could feel myself becoming discouraged with the way people behaved and what I had to deal with on a day-to-day basis. I can still picture in my mind, sitting in a police car on that estate thinking this is just a waste of time and then I became quite ill – I was depressed. I went to the doctor and he gave me some tablets, but things continued to get worse. The breaking point came one evening when I was sitting by myself in the police car. We were usually on our own as it was only a small place. I couldn't cope; I was in tears and I thought I couldn't do this anymore. The tablets took away my ability to function and I had to resign from the police force. I did not feel any purpose in life.

I managed to get a job in a parcel depot, first of all just shifting the parcels about before I became a driver. I was really low and I hit rock bottom; it was just dreadful. I was married with a child and a job without any thought of progress. I didn't know what I was doing or where I was going. I moved around like on automatic, just shifting these parcels around. That was about the lowest point that I reached. I didn't go back to the doctors then, and I didn't receive any more treatment.

This is where I met Rick, who had seen me struggling with life. He had noticed my depressive behaviour and my dreadful swearing (that's another military thing). Rick showed me compassion and became my friend, it meant so much at that point. I don't think I had many friends. I had my wife and family and I kept going for their sake, even though it was difficult. We were homeless for a while, which was hard. I had to live with my dad in a mobile home and my wife lived with her mum miles away; we were split up. When I managed to rent a dreadful property, it was cold and damp as the heating didn't work. We lived there until the council re-housed us, which helped a lot. I don't know what Rick thought, I mean, whatever he saw, he didn't treat me with disgust. This guy could see me coming unravelled, but I think because he'd been in a similar situation himself, he knew how difficult it was.

Rick also told me about Jesus, about my sins and

how Jesus died on the cross in my place. I listened to him. I found a little New Testament Bible that I got when I was in school. I worked at night, so I took my Bible to read at break time. The words that I read in the book of Revelation bothered me a lot. I couldn't stop thinking about them. Though, I couldn't wait to continue reading. One night, when I stopped for a break, I continued reading, and by then I realised that I was lost. I was a sinner in the eyes of God and deserved judgment. The Bible says that 'the wages of sin is death'. When I read the part that speaks about the new heavens and earth, I felt God's love flood over me and I knew what I had to do.

I closed the book and started driving down the road. I started to pray to Jesus, "I ruined my life, will you forgive me?" The answer was instant. I felt the weight of my sins lift from my shoulders, and a wonderful peace came to me. I was 'born again' I was forgiven and was now part of God's family. The next day I told my wife. She didn't understand. Two things stand out at this time. After a few days, I realised that I had stopped using foul language. Secondly, the words of the Bible came to life for me. I had a real hunger for the word of God. I had done things in my life that were not good, they were a great burden. So many burdens.

I started going to church. The Lord helped me a lot. Several years after my conversion, my wife was also saved. I wanted to serve The Lord and applied for a position with an organisation called 'The Soldiers and Airmen Scripture Readers Association (SASRA) as an army scripture reader. They are a ministry dealing with evangelism and pastoral outreach work in the forces. They wanted a scripture reader in my old regiment. The door seemed to be opening, then it was right in the middle of my application for the job that I started to feel unwell. I thought I had glandular fever. The disease intensified and the doctors had no answer. I had to stop my application to become a scripture reader. My world began to fall apart as the illness got worse and worse. The illness was diagnosed as myalgia encephalomyelitis - ME. It was the beginning of a long and difficult journey, but Jesus was with me all the time.

1991 was one of the most difficult years of my life. I was completely exhausted and could not continue. Where was God? Then it became worse! My sister, who lived in Portugal, was murdered. She had fought with her boyfriend who had beaten her to death with a shovel and dumped her body into a rubbish skip. I felt devastated and very low as I travelled to Portugal. She was my only sister and you never recover from something like that. People tell you that time heals but it doesn't.

Jesus went with me, and with the help of The Lord, I managed to find a good job in a local prison. My wife also worked there. I have worked with foreign nationals and illegal immigrants, and also as a resettlement officer for several years. It was a good time. I was also sometimes able to help in the Chaplain's department with Christian courses for prisoners. I had to leave this job in 2010 due to my ME illness.

The second of my most difficult times was in 2012 when my wife was taken ill with cancer. It was all very sudden whilst we were at Pilgrim's Hall retreat centre and she collapsed. She died just a few months later. The most difficult part came after she died and I started to sort through her stuff, I found that she owed thousands of pounds to people, including £12,000 to one of her best friends, it was like a punch in the stomach.

They talk about God's grace being sufficient and I found the strength to keep going. At that stage, I planned to buy Aspirin from various shops and bring an end to this horrible mess. I knew as a Christian that wasn't the right way to go and I don't think I would have ever done it, but I just said, "Lord, I can't do this anymore."

I didn't hear an audible voice, but I felt within my heart I had to go back to the church that I had previously been to with my late wife. The people there were great, and they were very kind; this is where I met Emma, my current wife. Before this, I would say that was about the lowest time of my life.

Fortunately, I had some money from the prison service, as my wife was a prison officer and she had died in service; I received a lump sum payment to help. I was able to pay off her debts, but it was just the shock of it all. I found bills, and County Court Judgments; all stuffed in bags, envelopes and in drawers under the table. I couldn't breathe and I was shaking. I went to Pilgrims Hall and one of the ladies, who was a nurse said, "Brian, you have post-traumatic stress, so go to the doctors." The doctor prescribed diazepam and something else. I could not deal with any more stress.

Living with ME has been a constant battle, from 1983 when I became ill to 1991. I'd had 15 jobs and lost them. It was like snakes and ladders, I would get well, I would climb up to the top of the ladder, then walk a few paces and I was down the snake. Each snake meant that I had to start again. In that year, 1991, I had a complete breakdown and thought this was too hard.

There have been times when my physical health improved and I even experienced a healing to a degree, but life has always been full of struggles. I've been housebound for about four years. I've lost count of the times that I've said, "I really can't do this." Then, I think of Jesus in the garden of Gethsemane and the thought that He didn't want to do that either. He didn't want to be in that place sweating great drops of blood knowing what was going to happen.

I often say to God, "I'm not having a bundle of laughs here, but not my will but yours." In all of my struggles, I can still see good things come out of them. Yet, there are too many Christians who think that we shouldn't be ill, especially mentally ill and there's this expectation in some people's minds that once you come to The Lord, you're great and you can skip through the flowers with a big smile on your face all day long, you have the victory and everything - We do but it's a hard life.

We need to notice those who are struggling and reach out to them. Rick kept at it and befriended me. He helped in practical ways as well, with little things. When we moved into our house the garden was a mess. Rick came and helped cut the grass and burn up the rubbish. It was bonfire night and he bought some fireworks and some people came around and we had a sort of bonfire night bash in the backyard. Showing that kindness made all the difference because he demonstrated compassion.

The Lord showed Rick what to do and it turned my life around. I had read many stories from people who had become Christians, as their lives had been falling apart. I recognised that when I worked in the prison service. I saw people turn to Jesus and let their lives transform.

During my working life I had very blokey jobs; army, police force, and prison service, I even worked for 5 years as a naval auxiliary. They were all very blokey and crying would be considered as being weak. However, I've been in such a depressed state that I could no longer cry, the tears dried up. I'd cried myself out of crying and everything went numb. Now I do cry again and I say, if you're struggling with stuff go somewhere and find a friend. If you haven't any friends, go somewhere to get some help. Go to a support group, don't just sit there and look for solutions in a bottle or in drugs or anything, you're not going to find it, it's going to make it worse. Find someone like Rick or be someone like Rick.

Dan's Story

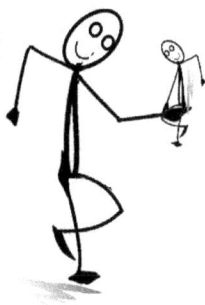

I'm an ex-army brat and I suppose the trauma all starts from moving houses. It was a constant upheaval, never really settled anywhere, that doesn't help with your mental health. That happened from a very young age and I find it difficult to explain some of my stories, they don't fit into a timeline because my memory has a great way of blocking out some of the past. Then suddenly things can just pop up out of the blue.

I always recall my parents never understanding other people and by that, I mean they didn't even understand their own parents. Why their parents behaved the way that they did? They were always falling out with friends and they fell out with their family, it was quite bizarre. My brother is super intelligent and they used to focus on his intelligence and compare him to me which wasn't so great. My sister had different needs, so again they would focus on that. They were hyper-focused on my brother who was up there and my sister who was down there and I was just Joe average in the middle but still with my own struggles. I'd always just get on with things so it is difficult to pinpoint when the trauma started but it's always been there.

I recognise the 'Black Dog,' an expression for depression, in my life. The other day I was struggling a little bit and I said you know he's there; he's nipping at my ankle. I recognise him and I can ask, "What am I going to do about it?" I'm never going to be your perfect picture; I don't think anyone is but I'm aware of where I am at and that is good. It's taken a long time to get there especially when my wife used to tell me all the time that I'm not very good. Over and over, I'm not very good. My response was, "Shut up! What do you know?"

The truth is that someone else usually knows you better than yourself and you don't want to know yourself because that's a painful side. I can now talk about my struggles and things, even though they have not gone but I'm in a good place at the moment. When I'm in a bad place, I simply say, everything's fine. 'Fine' is our favourite word, isn't it? We need to be honest when they ask that question, are you okay? It is okay to say, "No actually I'm having a really shit time today. Have you got 10 minutes for me?"

We often refer to going to dark places, I think this is a name that describes that which we don't want to talk about. We say our dark places but the truth is I wanted to kill myself. For me, the moment that I was at peace with wanting to kill myself was the time that it woke me up. That sounds bizarre but I was battling with it for a long time and then to reach a place of comfort, knowing I wanted to kill myself and I was comfortable with it. I wasn't worried about anyone else. I was comfortable and thought that they would be better off without me; that was a scary moment.

I was in that dark place for a long time and even now there's probably not a day that doesn't go by where I don't think about what it would be like. Even though I now support loads of people who are going through difficulties and I'm probably the go-to person if you need a little bit of motivation, there's probably not a week that goes by where I don't think I wonder what it would be like. It's not that I'm in a dark place, it's just that thought can still sit there. The old black dog is still sitting there, he's tamed now, he's not jumping up at me and clawing me with his muddy paws but he is still there.

A few years ago, I used to find it quite difficult. As well as carrying my own burdens, I also ended up carrying other people's burdens. I was a youth and community worker and, in the town where I live and work, several young people were taking their own lives. It was so bad that it did seem like every day. I would go into the office and wait to know which young person wasn't going to turn up for a club or which young person we would read about in a newspaper.

My full-time job is now helping people to move toward employment but I also volunteer for the Lads and Dads group. We can spend a lot of time just sitting and talking but for me, it's about sowing the seeds. This is more important than the harvest. I'll be sowing seeds and someone else can reap. To me, it's about people's self-belief, what they can do and those seeds of hope. Mindset is a big thing as well. I believe if you say that it's not going to happen then it probably won't; it's a simple self-fulfilling prophecy.

Good mental health is an essential aspect of our overall well-being, yet it remains a topic shrouded in stigma and misconception. For many years, I battled anxiety and depression silently, constantly worried about how it would impact my work and personal life. There is not a specific time in my life when I can say that symptoms of anxiety and depression began, as I believe I have always had trauma in my life since a young age. However, the darkest part of my life has been over the past 15 years. I left my first wife, which meant losing contact with my children. Soon after, I got married for the second time, and we lost a baby while she was pregnant. Within a few months of that, I found out I had cancer. Thankfully, after a few years and undergoing treatment, I was given the all-clear. Later, I reconnected with my daughter from my first wife, and she gave birth to my first grandson, who died just five days later.

Fearing the judgment and potential repercussions, I hid my struggles behind a mask, sacrificing precious moments with my loved ones and my happiness. I now aim to shed light on the stigma associated with mental health and emphasise the importance of seeking help and support.

Every day, I would return home from work drained, compelled to sleep away the exhaustion that anxiety and depression brought upon me. Weekends became an extended hibernation period, depriving me of precious time with my family. I missed my daughter's birthdays and Christmases, consumed by the weight of my inner turmoil. The fear of losing my job prevented me from seeking professional help, as I believed it would further jeopardise my already deteriorating mental state.

When I finally mustered the courage to visit a doctor, I was prescribed medication and put on a waiting list for additional support. Unfortunately, the support never materialised, leaving me feeling abandoned and further isolated. The impact of my mental health struggles extended to my relationship with my wife, who, overwhelmed by the challenges, asked me to leave. It was at this crucial juncture that I realised I needed to reach out for more help. Society often imposes rigid expectations on men, encouraging them to "grow up" or "man up" when it comes to mental health.

For many years, I did not want to admit that I had poor mental health. After a long time, I went to see the doctors and was given some pills, but they did not work. I took them for a long time. Then, I sought more support through counselling, but the waiting lists were long. I attended a 'Back to Work' group session, although I was already working. I thought it might help, but I cannot say whether it did or not. However, it triggered something in me that made me realise I needed to deal with this as I was drifting further away from my family. I wanted to be 'normal,' I wanted to be happy, and I wanted to enjoy family life. That desire was the start of my journey towards getting better.

However, I didn't know what to do or how to do it. I went to the doctors, and they gave me more pills and put me on more waiting lists. I paid for counselling, and that was the start of my recovery. I learned to talk about how I was feeling. My counsellor didn't have the answer to how to get better because the answer was within me. I decided to live on my own for a few years, and this pushed me to the edge. After going to the hospital to seek support, I decided no more pills and no darker places. I was going to change. I haven't taken a pill since, and now I feel like I have control over my mental health. I have done this with my mindset.

There exists a harmful stigma that portrays it as weak or shameful for men to acknowledge their struggles and ask for help. This stereotype only serves to perpetuate the silence surrounding mental health and prevents many from seeking the support they desperately need. The truth is that it is perfectly okay to ask for help and admit that you are struggling. It takes strength and courage to confront your mental health challenges head-on.

By breaking free from the chains of stigma, you open yourself up to the possibility of healing and growth. It is vital to remember that you are not alone in your journey, there are resources and support networks available to aid you. Employers have a crucial role to play in fostering a supportive work environment for individuals struggling with mental health issues. Promote open communication: Encourage a culture of open and honest communication where employees feel comfortable discussing their mental health concerns without fear of stigma or judgment. This can be done through regular check-ins, confidential channels for sharing concerns and promoting mental health awareness campaigns. Avoiding overwork and burnout can have a positive impact on employees' mental well-being. Encourage teamwork, collaboration, and positive relationships among colleagues. Provide training programs on mental health awareness and create spaces for open discussions.

Unfortunately, when I reached out to my workplace, no adjustments were made to accommodate my needs. This lack of understanding and empathy only exacerbated my challenges. Employers must recognise the importance of mental well-being and proactively offer resources, flexible work arrangements, and open communication channels to ensure their employees' holistic health.

Challenging the stigma surrounding mental health is a collective responsibility. It is imperative that we encourage open conversations, educate ourselves and others, and create safe spaces for individuals to seek help. Remember, it is more than okay to acknowledge your struggles, ask for help, and prioritise your mental well-being. In my workplace, I actively promote good well-being and mental health. Gone are the days when I would hide my own mental health challenges. Now, I openly share my experiences to help others.

Some final words of wisdom - I can't change the past that is the truth but you can use the past to be in the moment now and to make today amazing. You can't change tomorrow, that's the truth, you can only ever be in control of now, try focusing on what you've got rather than what you haven't. If you are in that dark place reach out, talk to someone before a cry for help becomes worse. I still battle every day with the echoes of my past and things that happened. Sometimes, it takes a lot more energy than running the marathon to get up in the morning but I get up and I fight.

An example of how Dan supports others

I remember the night vividly. It was 3 a.m. and I received a message, someone who I knew had been struggling for a while. The message was short, but I could sense the desperation in his words. He was not in a good place and needed someone to talk to. I knew that I had to act fast, so we exchanged a few messages back and forth to get a sense of the situation. It quickly became clear to me that he was on the verge of ending his life. I knew that I had to get up, get out, and go see him in person. I arrived at his house shortly after, feeling a mix of anxiety and determination. I knew that I had to be strong for him and provide the support that he needed. When I saw him, I could tell that he was not in a good place. He was in tears but relieved to see me. We spent a long time talking and listening to each other. I knew that I had to tread carefully, but also make sure that he knew he was not alone.

We talked through his feelings, and I encouraged him to seek professional help. Together, we made a plan of action. The waiting list for counselling was long, so we kept revisiting his goals and slowly but surely, he began to see the light. He went to see his doctor and we booked counselling sessions for him.

Over the next few months, I watched as he began to make progress. It wasn't easy, but he was determined to become the person he longed to be.

Here are some suggested coping mechanisms that you can adopt if you ever find yourself struggling to make progress towards becoming the person you long to be:

1. **Set Realistic Goals:** It's important to set achievable goals, so start with small and realistic ones. This way, you can build momentum and increase your confidence as you make progress.

2. **Practice Self-Care:** Taking care of yourself is crucial for your mental and emotional well-being. This includes eating healthy foods, exercising regularly, getting enough sleep and doing things that make you happy.

3. **Reach Out for Help:** It's okay to ask for help when you need it. Whether it's from a friend, family member, or mental health professional. Seeking support can make a huge difference.

4. **Challenge Negative Thoughts:** Negative thoughts can hold you back, so try to identify them and challenge them. Ask yourself if they are based in reality and if they are helpful or harmful.

5. **Practice Mindfulness:** Mindfulness is a technique that can help you stay focused on the present moment. It involves paying

attention to your thoughts, feelings and sensations without judgment.

6. **Build a Support System:** Having a support system can make a huge difference when you are struggling. This can include friends, family members and support groups.

7. **Learn from Setbacks:** Setbacks are a natural part of the journey towards personal growth. Instead of giving up, use setbacks as an opportunity to learn and grow.

Remember, making progress towards becoming the person you long to be is a journey, and it's important to be patient with yourself along the way.

Today, my friend is doing well. He still has his moments, but he knows where he wants to go and that he's not alone. It's amazing to see how far he's come and how much he's grown. I'm proud to have been there for him when he needed me most, and grateful that he trusted me enough to reach out for help. It's so important for friends, family, and loved ones to know how to reach out and offer support to those who may be struggling.

Here are some tips on how to start that conversation and end the stigma around mental health:

1. **Normalise the Conversation:** Start by normalising the conversation around mental health. Let your loved ones know that it's okay to talk about their struggles and that they are not alone. Share your own experiences and encourage them to do the same. But don't make it about you, after all, we are not all the same and we don't all deal with things in the same way.

2. **Show Empathy:** Show empathy towards your loved one's struggles. Try to understand their perspective and validate their feelings.

3. **Offer Support:** Offer support in any way that you can. This could be as simple as listening without judgment or helping them find resources and professional help.

4. **Educate Yourself:** Educate yourself on mental health and the resources available. This will help you better understand what they are going through and how to support them.

5. **Watch for Warning Signs:** Be aware of warning signs that someone may be struggling. This could include changes in mood, behaviour or habits.

6. **Encourage Professional Help:** Encourage professional help if needed. Offer to help them contact their doctor and support them on their journey towards achieving better mental health.

It's a reminder that sometimes, all we need is someone to listen, to understand, and to be there for us.

**Brendan Conboy has an active speaking
MINISTRY for GOD
And is looking forward to
hearing from you**

*Contact Brendan at the following:
Email – bmconboy@gmail.com
Phone - +44 (0)1453 731008
Mobile – 07980 404873
www.brendanconboy.co.uk*

**The following pages contain information
about Brendan's book titles (Bibliography).**

The Golden Thread – Biography
A true story of fear, forgiveness and faith
First published – 1ˢᵗ September 2015

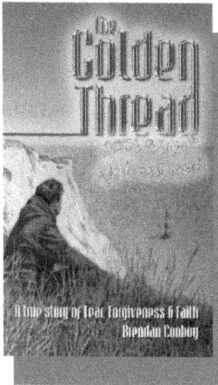

Brendan Conboy grew up in fear and confusion, struggling with many personal issues. These experiences formed a foundation that could have ended in disaster, but instead, became the motivator to want to make a positive difference.

Issues – Teen / YA Fiction
We all have issues… Can a bully change?
First published – 23ʳᵈ January 2019

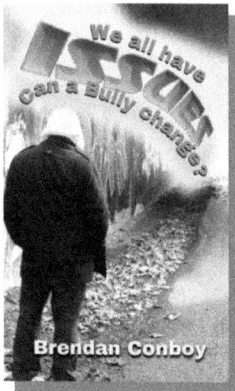

Marcus Daniel was a caring, intelligent, larger-than-average ten-year-old. His parents changed and then so did he. Now Marcus is thirteen years old and a spiteful bully, full of anger, rage and pain. His actions have changed others. Will the fear, pain and rage win?

My Foundation for Life – Semi Biog / Scriptural Teaching
14 underpinning and impacting scriptures
First published – 19th February 2019

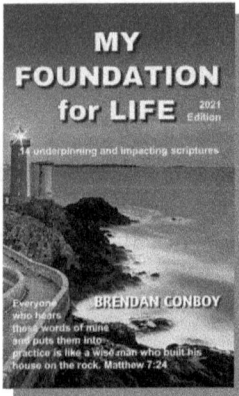

What is it that makes some of us more resilient than others? I am sure that psychologists will have several long-winded explanations to answer this question, but I believe that we can increase our resilience by building our lives on a foundation of truth

Rhyme Time – Poetry
Poems with a message for you to read.
Poems of truth that plant a seed.
First published – 13th November 2020

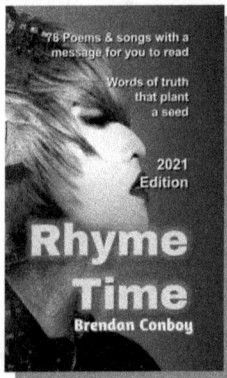

The Invasion of the Mimics
Science Fiction / Dystopian / Fantasy
They're already here… Invading your country…
Dwelling in your home… Living in your body!
First published – 21st October 2020

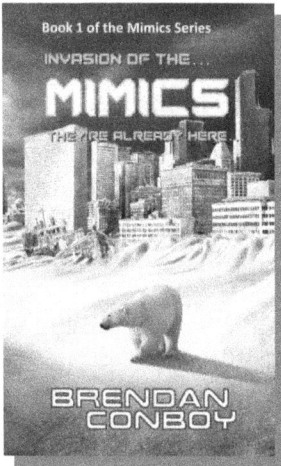

Climate change had been predicted long ago, but not one person could foresee the events that had unfolded. Humanity is defeated, civilisation lost, all hope has gone. Enlightenment is the new belief, but there are those who refuse to believe.

The Land of Make Believe – Children's fantasy in rhyme
Based on the story of doubting Thomas
First published – 4th March 2021

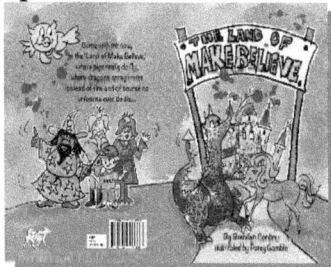

ONE GOD Many Names
First published – 14th July 2021

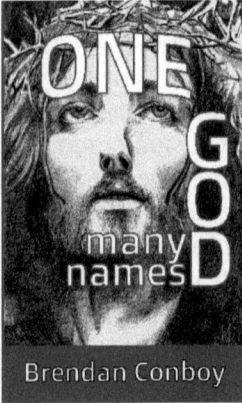

When we meditate on the many names of God, something powerful can happen to us. Brendan Conboy shares his thoughts and personal stories of what some of these names mean and how they had a transformational impact on his life.

The Book of PSALMS in Rhyme
First published – 24th August 2021

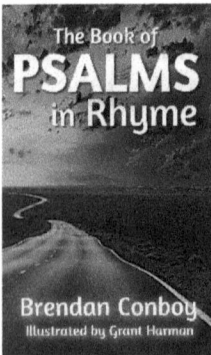

POWERFUL...
POETIC...

RHYTHMIC,
RHYMING
PSALMS...

A fresh expression to ignite your soul.

Legacy of the Mimics
First published – 20th June 2022

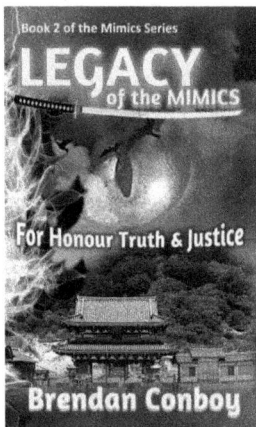

Book two in the Mimics series.
Her eyes told her everything was calm, as it should be. Her eyes deceived her. Her mind sensed something else.

Beyond the void

Popcorn Poetry
First published – 30th August 2022

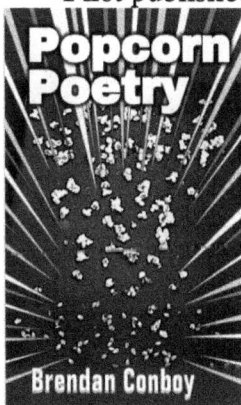

75 Poems that pop with rhythm & rhyme
The concept of **Popcorn Poetry** is simple, popcorn is made for sharing, just like the rhymes in this book - read them out loud and share them with friends.

Half Man Half Poet
First published – 2nd April 2023

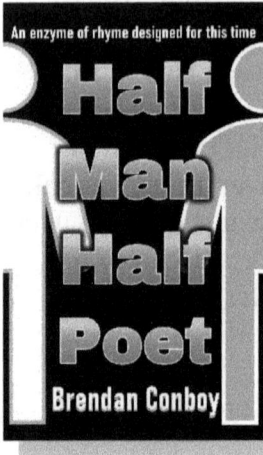

An enzyme of rhyme designed for this time
Life – Health – Social issues – Christian message. This book has something for everyone

The End is not The End
First published – June 2023

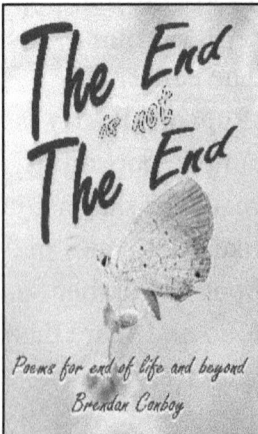

Poems for end of life and beyond – There is no avoiding death, it happens to us all. These poems will hopefully bring peace in the struggle.

The Gift
First published 25th September 2023

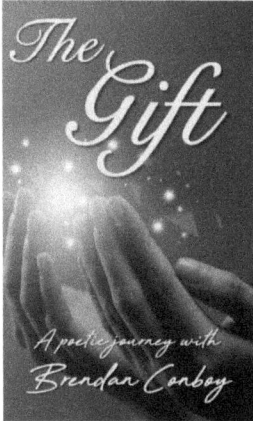

A compilation of four of my poetry books.

Rhyme Time

Popcorn Poetry

Half Man

The End

I'm Still Valued
First published – November 2023

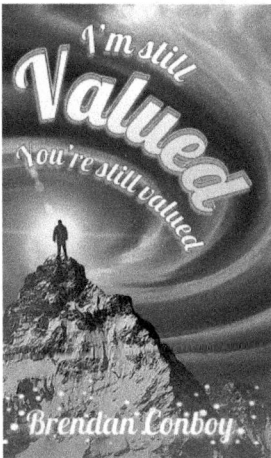

Brendan's continuing life story featuring a life-limiting and disabling kidney disease. He has faced many life-threatening battles and persevered. Almost died and been in the well-known, tunnel of light.

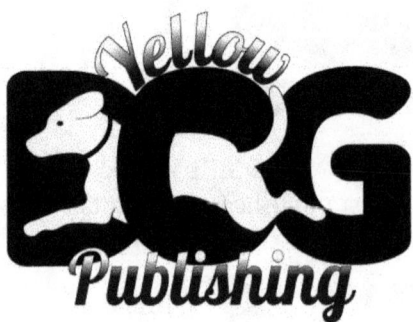
Yellow Dog Publishing

254